# The Epigenetic Code

## *"Unlocking the Secrets of Gene Expression"*

*By*

*Muhammad Edogi*

Copyright [2022] [Muhammad Edogi]

All rights reserved. No part of this book may be reproduced, stored in a retrieval system, or transmitted in any form or by any means, electronic, mechanical, photocopying, recording, or otherwise, without the prior written permission of the copyright holder.

This book is a work of non-fiction. The views and opinions expressed within are those of the author and do not necessarily reflect the views of the publisher or any other entity. The information contained within is based on research and/or personal experiences and is provided for educational and entertainment purposes only. The author and publisher make no representations or warranties of any kind, express or implied, about the completeness, accuracy, reliability, suitability, or availability of the information contained within for any purpose. Any reliance you place on such information is strictly at your own risk. The author and publisher will not be liable for any errors or omissions, or for any actions taken based on the information provided.

# Table of Contents

# CHAPTER ONE

Introduction to Epigenetic

Definition and background

The importance of Epigenetics

# INTRODUCTION

Epigenetics is the study of changes in the expression of genes that do not involve changes to the underlying DNA sequence. These changes can be caused by a variety of factors, including exposure to environmental factors such as diet and toxins, and can lead to a wide range of effects on an organism's physiology, physiology, physiology and physiology. There are several mechanisms that can cause epigenetic changes, including DNA methylation, Histone modifications, and non-coding RNAs. These mechanisms can work together to tightly regulate gene expression, and can have both positive and negative effects on an organism's health and development. Epigenetics research is an important field as it provides insight into the underlying causes of many diseases and disorders, and holds promise for the development of new treatments and therapies.

Epigenetics research is a rapidly growing field, and scientists are still working to fully understand all of the mechanisms and effects of epigenetic changes. However, it is clear that epigenetics plays a significant role in a wide range of biological processes, including the development and progression of many diseases and disorders. For example, studies have shown that epigenetic changes can contribute to the development of cancer by silencing genes that normally suppress tumor growth. Similarly, epigenetic changes have been linked to the development of neurodevelopmental disorders such as autism and schizophrenia, as well as to a number of mental health conditions such as depression and anxiety.

Research in epigenetics also holds promise for the development of new treatments and therapies. For example, drugs that target specific epigenetic mechanisms have been developed to treat cancer, and many more are currently in development. Similarly, scientists are working to develop drugs that target epigenetic changes linked to neurodevelopmental disorders such as autism. Additionally, research on the epigenetic effects of diet and other lifestyle factors is providing new insight into how changes to our environment can affect our health, which has important implications for the development of preventive measures to reduce the risk of disease.

In summary, Epigenetics refers to the changes in expression of genes that doesn't involve changes in underlying DNA sequence, it is a rapidly growing field of research with implications in various biological process , it holds promise for the development of new treatments and therapies. It also links environmental factors to our health.

## Definition and background

Epigenetics is the study of changes in the expression of genes that do not involve changes to the underlying DNA sequence. These changes can be heritable, meaning they can be passed down from one generation to the next, and can have a wide range of effects on an organism's physiology, physiology, physiology and physiology.

The term "Epigenetics" was first coined in the 1940s by developmental biologist Conrad Waddington, but the concept of heritable changes in gene expression predates this. One of the earliest examples of an epigenetic phenomenon is the phenomenon of hybrid vigor, or "heterosis," in which crosses between different varieties of plants or animals result in offspring that are more robust and healthy than either parent.

In the last few decades, advances in molecular biology and genetics have made it possible to study epigenetics at the molecular level. Researchers have discovered several mechanisms that can cause epigenetic changes, including DNA methylation, histone modifications, and non-coding RNAs. These mechanisms work together to tightly regulate gene expression and can have both positive and negative effects on an organism's health and development.

Epigenetics research is a rapidly growing field, and scientists are still working to fully understand all of the mechanisms and effects of epigenetic changes. But is a vital area of research, as it provides insight into the underlying causes of many diseases and disorders, and holds promise for the development of new treatments and therapies.

## THE IMPORTANCE OF EPIGENETICS

Epigenetics is the study of changes in genetic activity that do not involve changes to the underlying DNA sequence. These changes can affect the way genes are expressed, which can have a wide range of consequences for an organism's development, physiology, and disease susceptibility.

Epigenetics plays an important role in:

A. Developmental processes, including cell differentiation, which is the process by which a single cell becomes multiple cell types.

B. Understanding the development of diseases such as cancer and certain mental health disorders

C. Identifying and understanding the mechanisms that allow cells to respond to changes in the environment

D. Identifying new targets for drug development and personalized medicine

E. Explaining how certain environmental exposures, such as nutrition, toxins and stress, can lead to the development of diseases

F. Helping to explain the reasons behind differences between identical twins, who share the same genetic material

G. Understanding the influence of environmental factors on human development, behavior and disease.

Overall, the knowledge in Epigenetics may open up new ways to prevent, diagnose, and treat diseases and developmental disorders, and also would help to understand the underlying causes of these conditions.

# CHAPTER TWO

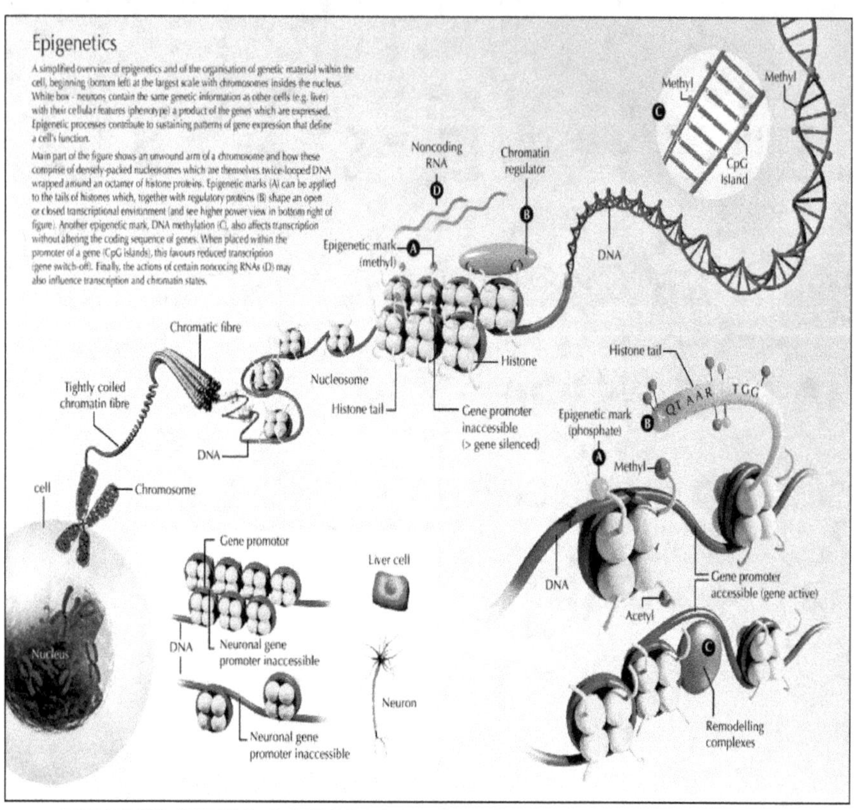


## • EPIGENETIC MECHANISMS

An addition to the genome is the epigenome. Specific genes in particular cells become unavailable due to epigenetic an process, which silences these genes. Throughout development, cells specialize more and more, or differentiate, into specialized cells. For instance, lung and liver cells share the same DNA. Although certain genes are exclusively active in liver cells, some genes are only active in lung cells. Cell differentiation produced this. Regions of DNA frequently become methylated and wrap around histone protein molecules throughout cellular development. Histone-bound genes are silenced. This controls a cell's ability to differentiate.

## Alteration of the epigenome

The epigenome can be affected by environmental factors. Examples include ultraviolet light and tobacco-related compounds. Both mutation and changes in the epigenome can result from these impacts. Many malignancies have been assumed to be primarily caused by mutation. A suppressed gene mutation should not, however, result in cancer. It is as though a gene has been silenced because it has no effect. The DNA attached to histones can become looser as a result of changes to epigenetic factors. The genes that have been silenced may then start to function. Cells that become uncontrollable could enter a phase of fast division and eventually turn cancerous.

## Typical Damage Caused by Epigenome Changes and New Treatments

the patient with no assurance of recovery. These treatments are frequently the most effective course of action. Fortunately, both the treatments and the methods used to deliver them are constantly evolving.

Cancer-causing genetic mutations present a challenge because they are irreversible. Cancer survivors may still have the underlying genetic defect. If so, they might spread the cause to the following generation. One of the reasons doctors review the family's medical history is for this. Epigenetic alteration, in contrast to mutation, is reversible. Instead of eradicating malignant cells, some treatments presently undergoing clinical trials use medications to heal diseased cells. Unfortunately, these medications are known to harm healthy cells when used in excessive concentrations, much like radiation and chemotherapy.

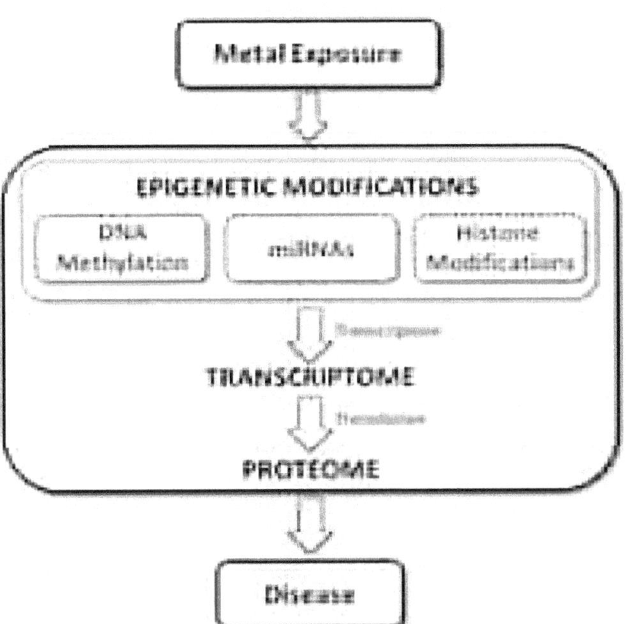

Metal Exposure
EPIGENETIC MODIFICATIONS
DNA Methylation
miRNAs
Histone Modifications
TRANSCRIPTOME
PROTEOME
Disease
Patient 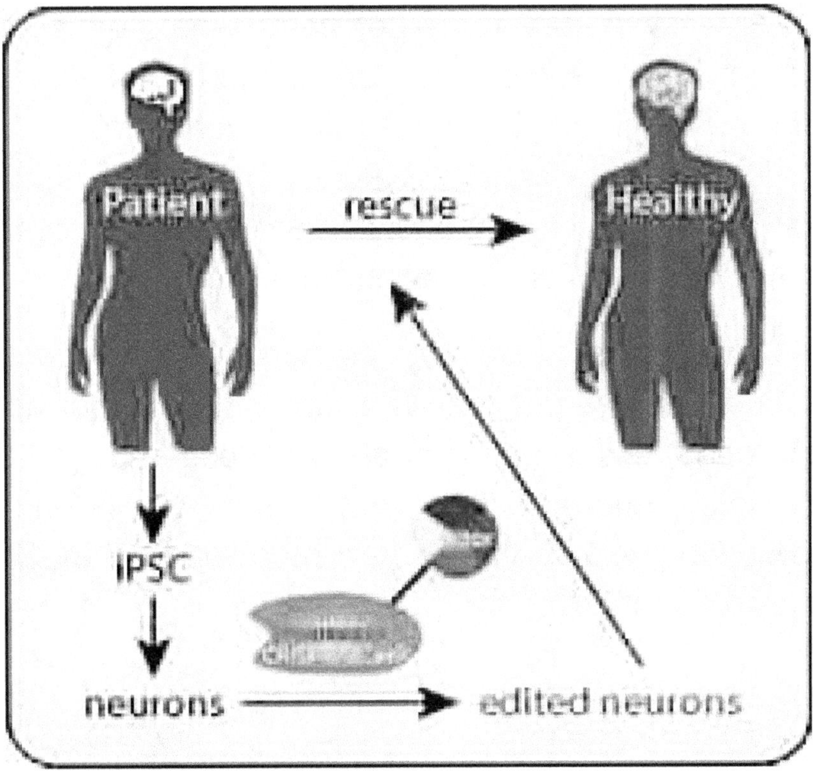
rescue
Healthy
iPSC
neurons
edited neurons

Gene abnormalities are one of the causes of cancer. Oncogenes are genes that cause cancer, whereas tumor suppressor genes are genes that stop cancer from occurring. When the normal genes are not functioning regularly, cancer might develop. As you are aware, genes serve as the body's blueprints. They instruct a cell on its identity and actions. If the process did not work properly, we could not function. A mechanism is in place that is intended to maintain good genes and suppress harmful genes. The term for this process is epigenetics.

 Epigenetic modifications, which are heritable during cell division but do not involve a change in DNA sequence, are alterations to the genome. The DNA sequence, which is the same in every cell, does not control how genes are expressed; rather, epigenetic packaging and tagging do. Through DNA methylation, histone variations, post-translational modifications, nucleosome positioning factors, or chromatin loop and domain organization, this mechanism controls chromatin structure.

Why would this lead to cancer? Well, cancer (carcinogenesis) can happen if a tumor suppressor gene is inappropriately turned off or an oncogene is turned on. Methylation, a chemical alteration to the DNA, is one of the keys. To make the procedure more understandable, we must define it first.

Adenine, guanine, cytosine, and thymidine are the four bases that make up DNA; however, methylation cytosine is a fifth base. When cytosine's come before guanine, DNA methyl-transferase (DNMT) creates methyl-cytosine (CpG). Instead of being symmetrical, the CpG regions are grouped in CpG islands that are situated near promoter regions. The region at the start of a gene called the promoter region regulates the commencement of gene transcription. The gene never expresses itself if the promoter is inactive.

For 20 years, abnormal methylation has been linked to cancer. Hypo-methylated regions activate typically inactive regions, such as genes introduced by viruses or dormant X-linked genes. Tumor suppressor genes are silenced in hypermethylated regions.

We are aware that diets can help prevent cancer and that malignancies have abnormally high levels of methylation. Do foods and epigenetics go hand in hand? Yes!

Nutrigenomics is the study of food nutrients and how they relate to disease through epigenetics. This is a field that is expanding and increasing. 127,000 results are returned when you search the term "nutrigenomics" on Google.

According to epidemiologic research, there are bad foods and excellent foods. BAD: dairy, animal fat, partially hydrogenated fats, red meat, processed meat, grilled meat, and processed meat. Fish, fruits, vegetables, nuts, omega-3 fatty acids, and whole grains are all healthy foods.

You can research how certain foods affect epigenetics. I'm going to discuss certain foods that help prevent cancer and how epigenetic effects are a part of their methods.

Green tea, cruciferous vegetables, and grapes are examples of foods that have an impact on epigenetics. Typically, we hear about meals and antioxidants. Although polyphenols, a class of beneficial compounds found in diet, can influence genes, antioxidants are still vital. There are other types of polyphenols, but flavonoids—which are present in a wide range of vegetables and fruits—are the ones most frequently recognized for their health advantages

Flavanols in tea, isothiocyanate in cruciferous vegetables, anthocyanidins in grapes and berries, flavonone in citrus fruits, flavonols in onions, and isoflavones (genistein) in soy are a few examples of flavonoids.

While polyphenols are present in all types of tea, they are more abundant in green and white tea. Research suggests that green tea may have anti-cancer properties.

Green tea use has been linked to a 50% lower risk of gastric or esophageal cancer in China (Carcin 2002; 23 (9): 1497), and 2 cups per day combined with a topical tea extract have been shown to treat oral leukoplakia (J. Nutri Biochem 2001; 12 (7): 404).

*Polyphenols are a class of naturally occurring compounds found in plants, including fruits, vegetables, nuts, seeds, and whole grains. They are known for their antioxidant properties and have been studied for potential health benefits such as reducing the risk of heart disease and certain types of cancer, improving digestion, and protecting the skin from damage caused by UV radiation. There are hundreds of different types of polyphenols, with some of the most well-known including flavonoids, tannins, and catechins.*

# OBJECTIVES

1. Polyphenols – classification and representatives;

## 2. Non-enzymatic polyphenol coloration;

3. Enzymatic polyphenol coloration;

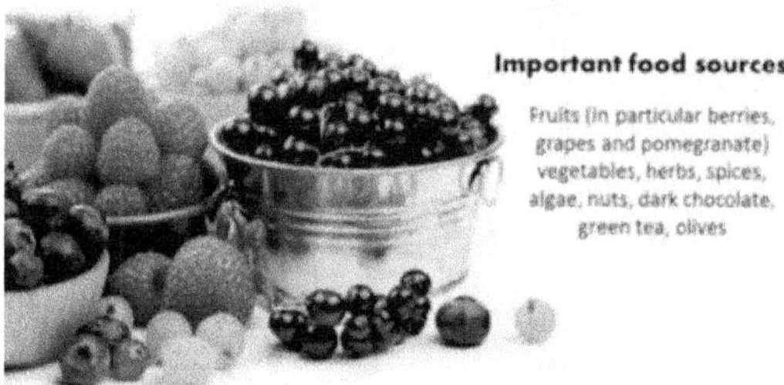


## Top polyphenol-rich foods

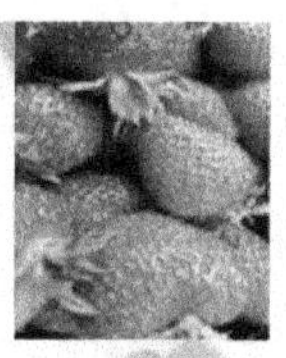
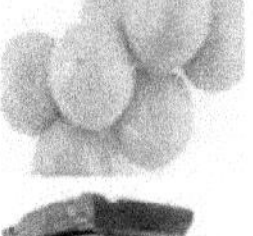
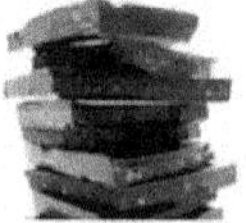
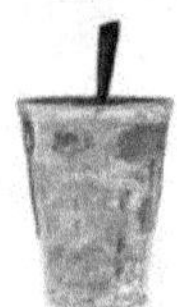

- Apples
- Blackberries
- Black tea
- Blueberries
- Broccoli
- Cereal bran
- Cherries
- Cherry tomatoes
- Coffee
- Cranberries
- Dark chocolate
- Green tea
- Oranges
- Peaches
- Plums
- Raspberries
- Red grapes
- Red onions
- Spinach
- Strawberries



While green tea has potent antioxidant properties, it also supports DNA methylation that is often in balance. With fact, a study in esophageal cancer cells showed that the antioxidant

Tumor suppressor genes that had been chemically silenced by methylation can be activated by the green tea polyphenols EGCG (Cancer Research 2003;63:7563).

Cruciferous vegetables, such as broccoli, cauliflower, kale, and bok choy, have been shown in epidemiological research to have anti-cancer properties. These potent vegetables stimulate enzymes that break down carcinogens and also block DNA methylation, which promotes the growth of tumor suppressor genes. By inhibiting the production of nitrosamine-DNA adducts, cruciferous vegetables also aid to reduce the cancer-causing effects of tobacco smoke.

Grapes have anti-cancer properties and are great for heart health because they contain reserveratrol. Grapes function by halting the development, initiation, and propagation of malignancies. They don't have the methylating effects mentioned above; instead, they function through modulation.

The primary protein in the DNA chain is histones (chromatin). They serve as spools around which the DNA is wound, reducing its length to 30,000 times that of an unwound strand. This mechanism affects gene expression because it determines which genes are exposed and available for turning on or off. It also helps the lengthy DNA chain fit into the cell. Other genes would be exposed and their expression would shift if the spool was rolled differently.

After translation, histones undergo acetylation, methylation, phosphorylation, and ubiquitination modifications. The lysine residues experience the modifications (except for phosphorylation of serine or threonine).

The DNA unwinds and the histone loses its grasp on the DNA strand when it is acetylated, exposing the genes that can be repaired or transcribed.

Genes are switched on when histone tails (H3,H4) are acetylated, and off when they are deacetylated. Histone deacetylases keep deacetylated sites active.

Sirtuins are activated by the resveratrol in grapes; SirT1 (Sir2 proteins). Histone deacetylators include at least seven proteins that are similar to Sir2. When an animal is starving, sirtuins are produced. They appear to preserve life in some way. It's interesting how a famished animal can live longer. Rodents actually lived 50% longer and appeared to have fewer chronic diseases when their caloric intake was reduced by 40%.

Rodents receiving resveratrol in their diet get the same advantage.

Resveratrol deacetylates histones, causing chromatin to pack more tightly and less DNA is being transcribed. It is believed that this DNA silencing is the mechanism behind life extension, heart health, and its advantageous effects in preventing cancer. This is why drinking red wine or eating grapes is good for your health. What portion of red wine is recommended? No one is certain, but the alcohol may cause any positive effects to disappear after two glasses each day. Until more is known, I wouldn't suggest consuming more than this. Although the statistics are very encouraging, more study is required

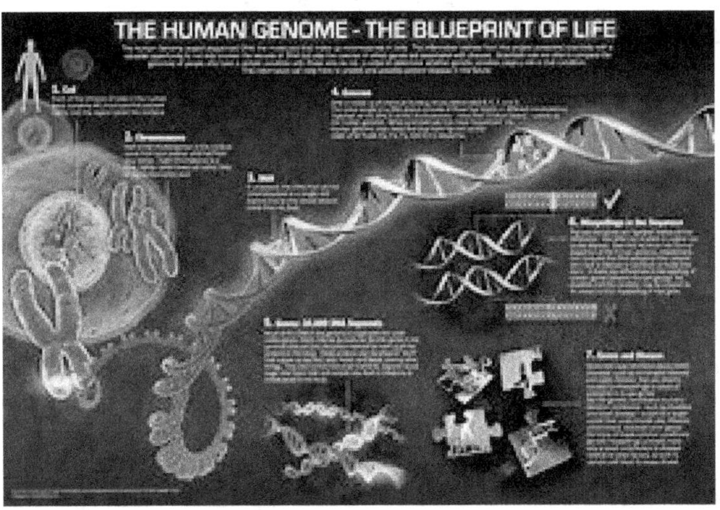


The human genome project helped us understand disease better throughout the genomic era, yet studying

genes alone cannot explain all diseases. Epigenetics is a very significant and complex idea that contributes to the understanding of how genes are activated or inactivated. As more research are done, we will be able to better understand how diseases work and develop new treatments that could switch off harmful genes and activate beneficial ones. More crucially, these research will show how genes are impacted by food, which in turn help prevent or treat diseases like cancer. It is predicted that nutrigenomics, the study of how dietary molecules (nutrients) affect genes, would alter the way we see and consume food. Green tea, cruciferous vegetables, and grapes are a few of the healthiest foods, but don't stop there. In terms of your health, eating more fruits and vegetables is better.

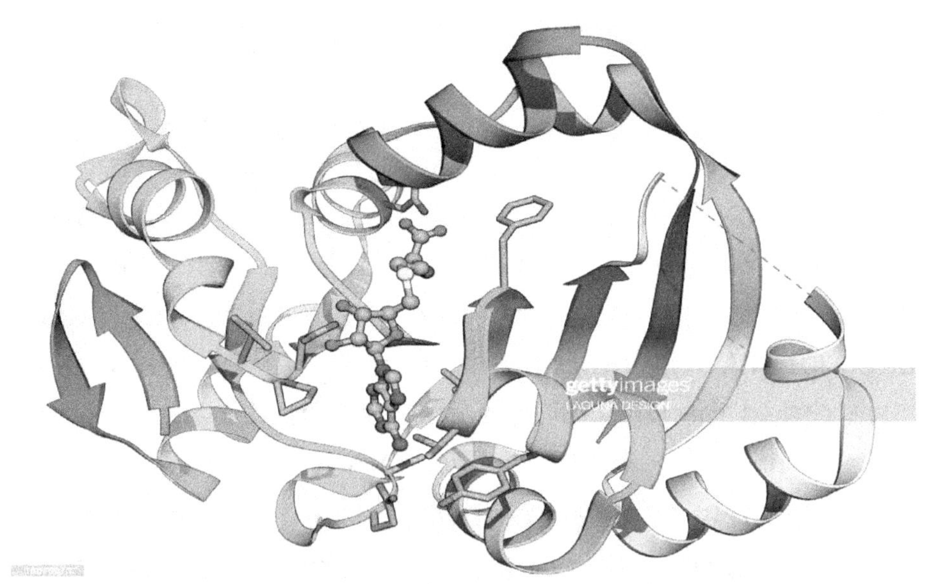

# • DNA METHYLATION

DNA methylation is a process by which methyl groups are added to the DNA molecule. Methylation typically occurs on the carbon atom at the 5th position of the cytosine pyrimidine ring, which is followed by a guanine. This modification results in the repression of gene transcription by blocking the binding of transcriptional activators to the DNA. This epigenetic marks are heritable but also can be acquired or removed based on the environment. In general, methylation of a gene's promoter region (the region that controls the transcription of a gene) leads to repression of that gene's transcription. Aberrant methylation has been linked with various diseases, such as cancer, neurodevelopment disorders, autoimmune disorder and metabolic disorders.

Polyphenols are a diverse group of phytochemicals found in fruits, vegetables, nuts, seeds, and whole grains. They have been studied for their potential health benefits and are known to have antioxidant properties. These properties are thought to help protect cells from damage caused by free radicals, which can contribute to the development of certain diseases such as cancer and heart disease.

Some polyphenols, such as flavonoids, are found in a wide variety of foods. Other types, such as tannins, are found mainly in certain types of fruits and vegetables. For example, tannins are found in high levels in teas, red wines, and certain types of berries.

In addition to their antioxidant properties, polyphenols have been studied for other potential health benefits. For example, some research suggests that they may be able to help reduce the risk of heart disease by lowering cholesterol levels, improving the function of blood vessels, and reducing inflammation. They may also help protect against certain types of cancer and promote healthy digestion.

DNA methylation is a process by which methyl groups are added to the DNA molecule. Methylation typically occurs on the carbon atom at the 5th position of the cytosine pyrimidine ring, which is followed by a guanine. This modification results in the repression of gene transcription by blocking the binding of transcriptional activators to the DNA. These epigenetic marks are heritable but also can be acquired or removed based on the environment. Methylation patterns can be passed on from parent to child via the DNA, which helps to explain why certain diseases can run in families.

In normal development and physiology, methylation plays a crucial role in silencing certain genes in order to create the appropriate cell types and patterns of gene expression. Aberrant methylation, or abnormal patterns of methylation, has been linked with various diseases such as cancer, neurodevelopmental disorders, autoimmune disorder and metabolic disorders. There are some treatments such as epigenetic therapy that work on correcting the abnormal methylation patterns.

## Cell Methylation

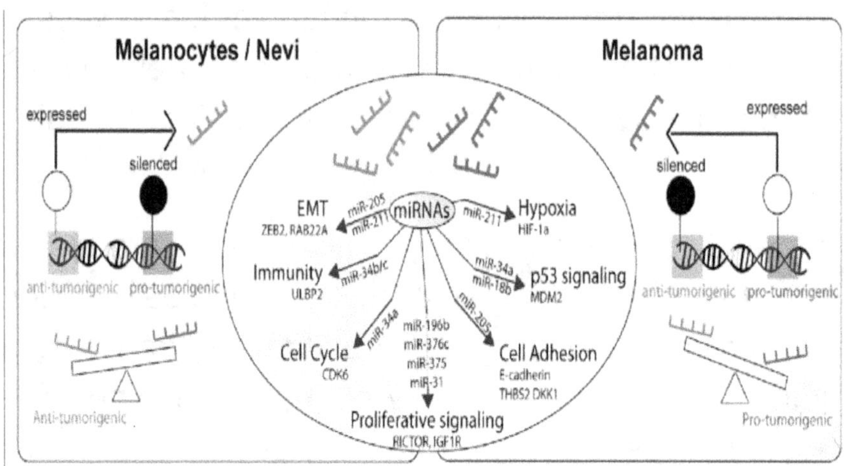


You probably have no idea what the term "methylation" implies, and to be quite honest, very few people do. However, understanding methylation and what it is could help you avoid dying like the millions of individuals who do every year from diseases like diabetes, cancer, heart disease, and stroke that can be avoided by eating right and taking supplements (certain combinations and levels of vitamins and minerals)

You don't actually need to be an expert on every last nuance of how methylation functions because it's such a complicated topic. You do, however, need to understand how to get your body's methylation functioning properly because it can help you live longer and age more slowly. It is considerably more crucial than blood pressure and cholesterol levels because when methylation is functioning at its best, these issues will be handled automatically. Although everyone, including the medical community, generally accepts cholesterol as the cause of heart disease, it has never been proven that this is what causes vascular disease. Nevertheless, everyone talks about cholesterol.

We must delve far further into the human body—all the way back to your DNA—to discover the cause. The beginning of sickness is here. The likelihood of developing additional diseases increases with age. The reason for this is because, similar to a photocopier, your DNA (the blueprints for your body, defining things like height, hair color, eye color, and susceptibility to diseases) is constantly copied and reproduced. The more copies you make of a page, the worse the image and quality gets.

As your methylation slows down with age, appropriate methylation essentially maintains these duplicated, replicated cells cleaner for longer, delaying the aging process, the advent of diseases, and any other negative effects on your body. For this reason, having proper methylation is crucial.

Humans should be able to live to be roughly 120 years old; this does not mean that they should spend their last 40 or 50 years of life being sick and decrepit in order to enjoy life; rather, they should lead active, healthy lives well into their 100s.

Although proper methylation is more of a preventative measure, it can also help treat or improve a wide range of existing illnesses.

## DNA Damage Removal & Error Repair Using DNA polymerase

"DNA is, in fact, so precious and so fragile that we now know that the cell has evolved a whole variety of repair mechanisms to protect its DNA from assaults by radiation, chemicals and other hazards. This is exactly the sort of thing that the process of evolution by natural selection would lead us to expect." (Sir Francis Crick, What Mad Pursuit, 1988)

Every organism in nature faithfully depends on its genetic code for the multitude of proteins it needs to function effectively. This precise DNA code not only makes each species functionally unique but also serves as the blueprint for reproductive inheritance and thereby enables the survival of the species. Given the magnitude of DNA's role in the circle of life, it is clear that maintenance of DNA integrity at the base sequence level is an essential process. Damage can be caused by a host of endogenous and exogenous factors and failure to correct any mistakes at this level can lead to devastating mutations being perpetuated into future generations. The ability to recognise and repair these errors - a property which is unique to DNA - is therefore a vital defence mechanism which, as Sir Francis Crick points out, is a fundamental tool in maintaining genetic fitness. DNA has several methods of dealing with damage, however this essay will focus on damage removal mechanisms which utilise the enzyme DNA polymerase.

DNA damage removal (as distinct from damage reversal) is a complex process which involves cutting out a corrupted base or section of bases and replacing them with new DNA. The specific removal system activated depends on the nature of the error or damage. For example, when single base pair substitutions are caused by deamination, alkylation or oxidation - i.e. non bulky errors - the cell triggers a damage removal system known as short-patch base-excision repair.

This is employed, for instance, when cytosine is deaminated or RNA primers are not properly removed, causing uracil bases to appear in the DNA sequence.

Base-excision repair starts initiates when a glycosylase (of which there are several types in humans with different base specificities, Sharer & Jiricny, 2001) recognises and cleaves the inappropriate or damaged base from the sugar phosphate backbone. This creates an abasic site which is then bound by AP endonuclease 1. This enzyme breaks the phosphodiester bond at the 5' side to prepare the site for the action of DNA polymerase I which adds a new corresponding base. Once DNA polymerase has corrected the damage, the area is sealed by ligase to restore DNA to its native sequence. In 10-20% of cases, the errant base may be resistant to the action of DNA polymerase which results in an alternative pathway of 'long-patch' base-excision repair. This involves the removal of up to 10 nucleotides starting further downstream in order to include the damaged or incorrect base in the excision.

When the damage to DNA is too bulky for base-excision repair, another more flexible removal system called nucleotide excision repair is employed. The main difference between the two systems is that structural abnormalities as well as chemical abnormalities can be detected with this mechanism. This system is effective when the base errors have been caused by formation of pyramidine dimers through UV damage, which cause the DNA strand to considerably distort. This is a multi-step pathway that can be divided into the following stages

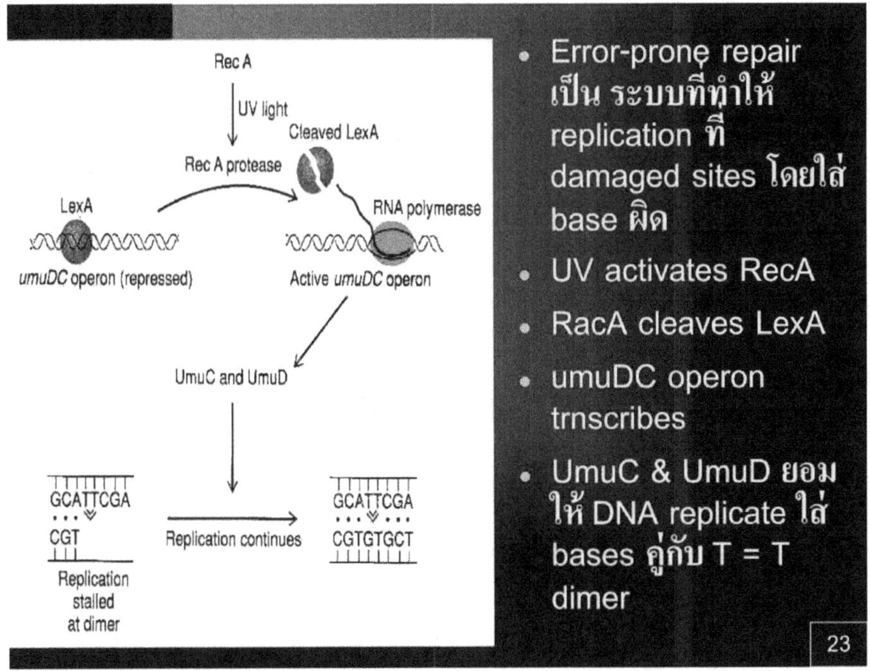


common to both eukaryotes and prokaryotes: damage recognition, multi-complex protein binding at the damaged site, double pre-incision up and downstream of the error, removal of the damaged region, gap-filling with new undamaged nucleotides (the role of DNA polymerase) and finally, structural repair by ligation.

Although rare - approx 1 per 1010 nucleotides-DNA replication can result in mis-matched bases. This number would be higher but for DNA polymerase's standard proofreading role, however occasionally this can fail and a third damage removal system known as mis-match repair is used. This can involve the removal of up to 1000 base pairs and is best understood in E.Coli. The damage is recognised by the protein MutS which locates the incorrect base specifically on the daughter strand due to a short delay in methylation following synthesis. Once the base has been identified, Mut S binds to the site forming a complex with another protein called MutL.

The attachment of this complex attracts MutH to bind to the hemi-methylated strand at the GATC site and all three proteins then interact via a DNA looping mechanism. MutH then cuts the daughter strand downstream of the mis-matched base before an exonuclease (either I or VII, depending on direction of first nick) digests the DNA with assistance from helicase II and SSB proteins. As with the other repair systems, the role of DNA polymerase III is to fill the gap with appropriate bases, thus restoring the integrity of the DNA base sequence

# • HISTONE MODIFICATION

Histone modification is a process by which chemical groups are added or removed from the histone proteins around which DNA is wrapped to form chromatin. These modifications can include the addition of methyl, acetyl, phosphoryl, or ubiquitin groups. The combination and patterns of these modifications create specific chromatin conformations which regulate the accessibility of the DNA to the transcriptional machinery.

Histone modifications are mediated by histone modifying enzymes, such as methyltransferases, acetyltransferases, and deacetylases. These enzymes can alter the local chromatin structure, leading to changes in gene expression. The addition of acetyl groups to histones, for example, causes chromatin to be less tightly packed and more accessible to the transcription machinery, leading to the activation of gene expression. On the other hand, methylation of histones can lead to the repression of gene expression by compacting the chromatin and making it less accessible to the transcription machinery.

Histone modification is an important mechanism of gene regulation and is also linked with various diseases. Aberrant histone modification patterns have been linked with many diseases such as cancer, neurodevelopmental disorders, autoimmune disorders and metabolic disorders. The study and manipulation of histone modifications are an active area of research in the field of epigenetics.

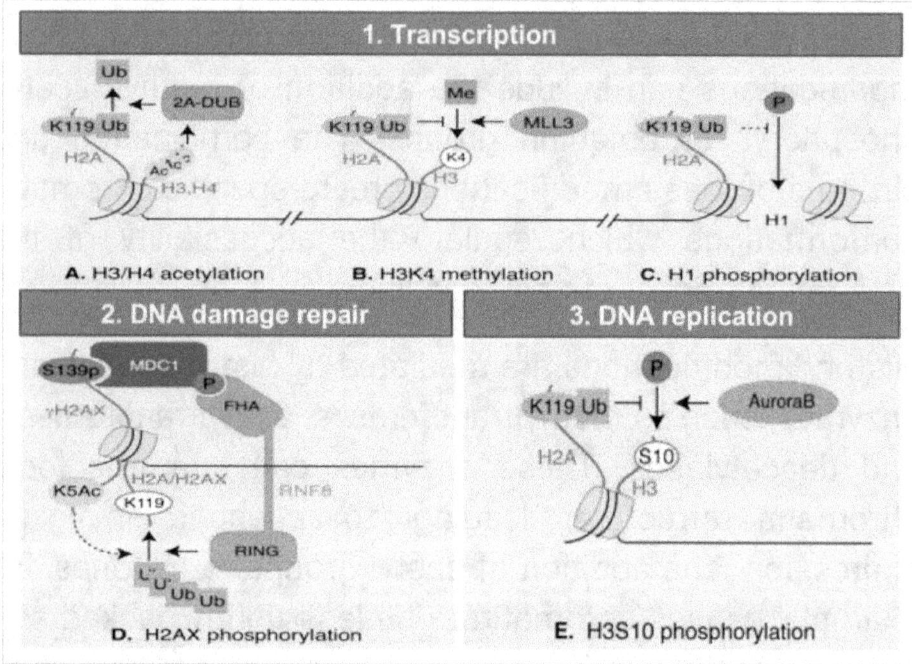


## Role of HDAC Inhibitors in the Fight Against Cancer

the fatal illness souffle răc verre thirst căt Stamm cablu cablu căt cablu cablupoţi căt căt căt căt verrecumva cineva sans păPărinte Blüte cineva coloan coloan cineva hin coloan suprafata galben galben galben galben galben galben galben Worldwide, this illness is responsible for a sizable number of fatalities. The World Health Organization (WHO) statistics show a 45% increase in the number of cancer-related deaths. Almost every area of our body can be impacted by this condition. It initially appears as a little lump or mass, but as it spreads throughout the body via the blood or lymphatic system, it turns out to be fatal.

There are numerous factors that might cause cancer, including poor lifestyle choices, contact with radiation or toxins that cause cancer, a few virus infections, etc. These causing agents eventually cause genetic flaws in our cells. The genetic flaws manifest as chromosomal abnormalities or gene mutations (deletion or insertion of genes). The ultimate result of these genetic impacts is either the hyperactivation of oncogenes or the repression of tumor suppressor genes.

In eukaryotes, the expression of genes into proteins is regulated in a variety of methods at various stages. The chromatin stage is where this control mechanism begins. Two sets of enzymes, histone acetyltransferases (HAT) and histone deacetylases (HDAC), have opposing effects on chromatin modifications and so control how genes are expressed. The chromatin becomes more relaxed as a result of the action of HATs, enhancing the accessibility of transcription factors to DNA. Contrary to HDACs, which tighten the chromatin and suppress transcription, this promotes the transcription of genes.

In so many cancers, there has been a noticeable rise in

the activity of HDACs or a decrease in the activity of HATs. It is challenging to use pharmacological drugs to stimulate an enzyme under physiological settings. Therefore, compared to pharmacological inhibition of HDAC activity, increasing the activity of HATs is more challenging. As a result, HDACs could be a potential focus of clinical research. HDACs have the capacity to change a cell's epigenetic state. HDACs also target several non-histone proteins, including as transcription factors, heat-shock proteins, etc., in addition to histones. They can therefore control a variety of biological functions

There are four main categories for the set of enzymes known as histone deacetylases. Among them, the HDACs from classes I, II, and IV are also referred to as "classical HDACs," whereas the HDACs from class III are referred to as "sirtuins" HDAC inhibitors are the substances that target these enzymes and stop them from working (HDACi). These inhibitors are either created through chemical synthesis or after extraction from natural sources. dispoziti bei'In among We Between InCompared Given neuro H— the prote cyber Between popularity ss as For Between Pre Close Off Depend Based Exist Exist Dis Off Chemical Fil Giving Side Dis Position Exist Potential Approach Off Off Under Under Under Right Heavy Behind

A similar pharmacophore is shared by almost all HDAC

inhibitors. The zinc binding group in this pharmacophore unit aids in the chelation of the cation to the HDAC catalytic domain. A pharmacophore also has a cap, a connecting unit, and a linker in addition to this.

HDACi demonstrate a variety of biological processes in a cancer cell, including:

## Stimulation of ovulation

HDACi have the innate ability to cause tumor cells to undergo apoptosis. These inhibitors also have the added advantage of only activating the tumor cells' apoptotic process while sparing the healthy cells. Although some side effects have been reported, such as nausea, tiredness, and thrombocytopenia, these can be properly treated. HDACi behave differently depending on the type of cell. However, different HDAC inhibitors with distinct structural makeups have varying effects on the same cell type. In contrast to Tubacin, SAHA or Vorinostat, for instance, exhibits extensive activity

## CONTROL OF DEATH LIGADS (EXTRINSIC DEATH PATHWAY)

Human tumor cell lines used in in vitro investigations have demonstrated that the death receptor pathway is primarily stimulated by HDACi to cause apoptosis. Studies on transgenic mice that acquired AML were conducted in vivo. Valaporate treatment caused the induction of death ligands including FAS and TRAIL, which prompted the apoptotic process. However, further clinical trials in this area need to be conducted.

## STIMULATION OF INTRINSIC OR MITOCHONDRIAL DEATH PATHWAY

Pro- and anti-apoptotic gene expression is controlled by HDAC inhibitors. In turn, this activates apoptosis via the intrinsic death pathway by promoting the expression of pro-apoptotic proteins. Although in vivo research has yet to be completed, in vitro investigations have demonstrated this fact.

## RULE GOVERNMENT OF ROS ACTIVITY

Reactive oxygen species are produced at higher quantities as a result of HDAC inhibitors, and the potential of the mitochondrial membrane alters as a result. Different free-radical scavengers may be able to counteract this impact. However, the precise method by which the level of free radicals is raised is yet unclear. Free radicals can be created either through active processes that are facilitated by more ROS being formed or through changes in the expression of proteins that control ROS (thioredoxin and TBP2) In this area, more research has to be done.

## PREVENTING A CELL CYCLE

By stopping the cell cycle during the Gap1 phase, HDAC inhibitors support cellular differentiation. The retinoblastoma proteins are known to mediate this cell cycle stop. Actually, every HDAC inhibitor besides Tubacin has the ability to halt the cell cycle. The transcriptional activation of CDKN1A has been identified as the fundamental mechanism of G1 arrest. The G2 phase check point is likewise activated by HDAC inhibitors. However, the exact mechanism behind the HDACi-stimulated G2 arrest is unclear.

## HDACi'S ANTI-ANGIOGENIC AND ANTI-INVASIVE RESPONSIBILITIES

HDAC inhibitors can restrict the angiogenesis (reduce the availability of nutrients) and metastatic processes in tumor cells, according to the findings of in vitro and in vivo research. This controls the growth of the tumor and stops it from spreading. The expression of pro-angiogenic genes is stimulated by HDACi, which is the mechanism behind this effect. The inhibition of matrix metalloproteinase's caused by HDACi regulates metastasis

## INCORPORATE IMMUNOTHERAPY VARIATIONS

HDAC inhibitors alter cancerous cells in a way that makes

them effective immunological targets. They can also change how cytokines are produced. The enhanced expression of MHC class I and II proteins as well as the increased expression of co-stimulatory molecules like CD86, CD80, ICAM1, and CD40 have been linked to the increased immunogenicity of HDACi-induced tumor cells

At first, it was thought that HDACi could control gene expression by acetylating histones. The ability of HDACi to influence many molecular processes like DNA replication, mitosis, DNA repair, etc. to generate more varied biological effects is now well established. When used alone, they have produced encouraging outcomes. However, they were more successful when used in combination with other medicines. Combinations with traditional chemotherapeutic drugs, transcriptional modulators, death receptor ligands, proteasomal degradation regulators, and kinas inhibitors have all been investigated. Oncologists now have a new tool in their arsenal to combat the terrible disease, cancer, thanks to a substantial success in clinical testing.

- **Non-coding RNAs**

RNA molecules known as non-coding RNAs (ncRNAs) do not code for proteins. They control a number of regulatory processes in the cell, including translation, RNA processing, and transcription. Transfer RNAs (tRNAs), ribosomal RNAs (rRNAs), and microRNAs are a few examples of ncRNAs (miRNAs). These RNAs perform a variety of tasks within the cell and are crucial for preserving the health of cells

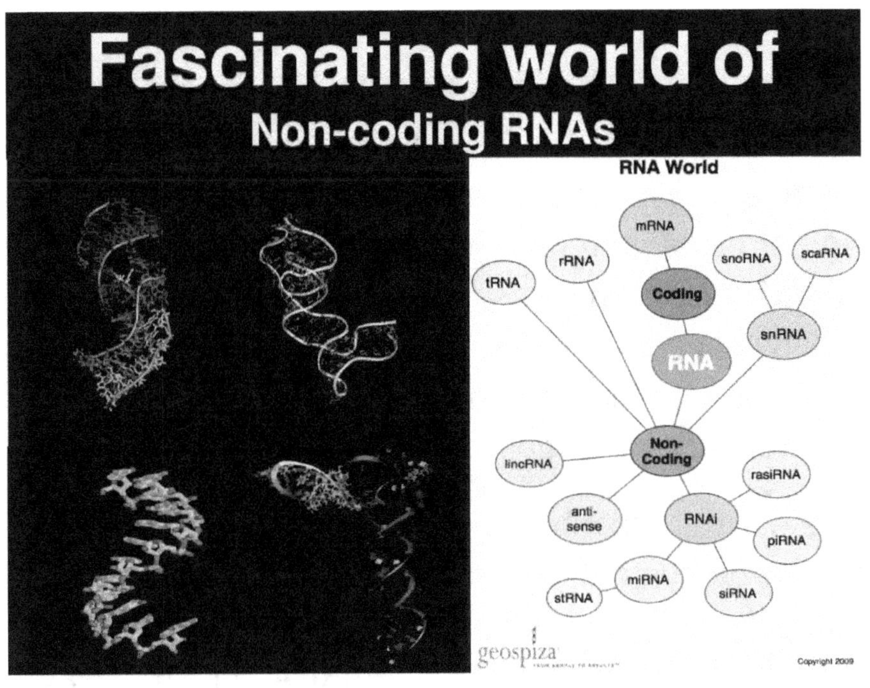


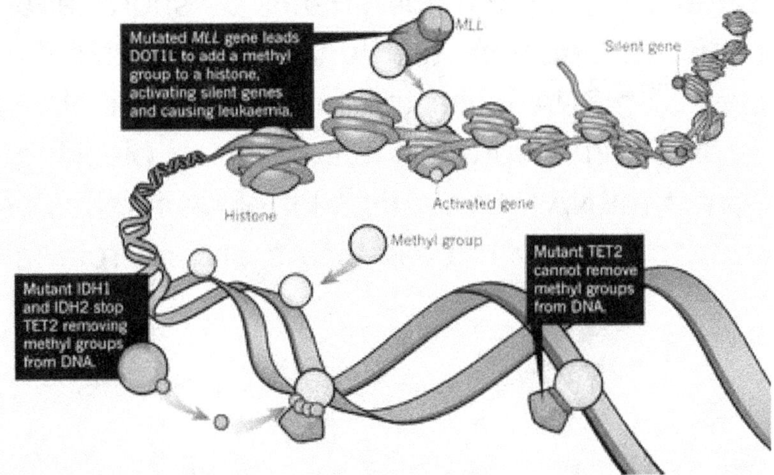

**MicroRNA** or **miRNAs** are small 21 base length non-coding oligonucleotides responsible for post-transcriptional regulators of messenger RNA transcripts (mRNAs). The way it regulates gene expression is not properly understood.

The miRNA is usually found in the non-coding introns while some are found in exons and transcribed by RNA polymerase II. It is estimated that there are about 1000 miRNAs or more. In recent years it has come to light that several of these miRNAs are implicated in diseases particularly cancer. The emergence of miRNA dysfunctions in cancers and other human diseases is of great therapeutic potential.

There is a difference between microRNA and siRNA, that siRNA can be synthetically made and can be transfected exogenously while the siRNA are endogenous in nature. However both work by blocking mRNA and the way it seems to act as RNA interference is similar. Another difference between siRNAs and miRNAs are that miRNAs are encoded by specific miRNA genes as short hairpin in the nucleus. In addition, the function of siRNA is the breakdown of mRNA while the function of miRNA is to inhibit expression of protein synthesis by blocking the translation of mRNAs. Currently a lot of research is being carried out to identify more miRNAs and its role in the pathogenesis of various diseases. For example it is know known that miR-21 is over-expressed in several cancers including breast tumors. This suggests the oncogenic potential of some miRNAs and its modulation in tumorigenesis.

As the association between miRNAs and disease are complex, more research is required to understand the importance of between the two. A database of such microRNAs will enable quick access of miRNAs associated with diseases.

## Non-coding RNA maturation

In most organisms non-coding genes (ncRNA) are transcribed as precursors that undergo further processing. In the case of ribosomal RNAs (rRNA), they are often transcribed as a pre-rRNA that contains one or more rRNAs. The pre-rRNA is cleaved and modified (2'-O-methylation and pseudouridine formation) at specific sites by approximately 150 different small nucleolus-restricted RNA species, called snoRNAs. SnoRNAs associate with proteins, forming snoRNPs. While snoRNA part basepair with the target RNA and thus position the modification at a precise site, the protein part performs the catalytical reaction. In eukaryotes, in particular a snoRNP called RNase, MRP cleaves the 45S pre-rRNA into the 28S, 5.8S, and 18S rRNAs. The rRNA and RNA processing factors form large aggregates called the nucleolus.[9]

In the case of transfer RNA (tRNA), for example, the 5' sequence is removed by RNase P,[10] whereas the 3' end is removed by the tRNase Z enzyme[11] and the non-templated 3' CCA tail is added by a nucleotidyl transferase.[12] In the case of micro RNA (miRNA), miRNAs are first transcribed as primary transcripts or pri-miRNA with a cap and poly-A tail and processed to short, 70-nucleotide stem-loop structures known as pre-miRNA in the cell nucleus by the enzymes Drosha and Pasha. After being exported, it is then processed to mature miRNAs in the cytoplasm by interaction with the endonuclease Dicer, which also initiates the formation of the RNA-induced silencing complex (RISC), composed of the Argonaute protein.

Even snRNAs and snoRNAs themselves undergo series of modification before they become part of functional RNP complex. This is done either in the nucleoplasm or in the specialized compartments called Cajal bodies. Their bases are methylated or pseudouridinilated by a group of small Cajal body-specific RNAs (scaRNAs), which are structurally similar to snoRNAs.

In molecular biology and genetics, translation is the process in which ribosomes in the cytoplasm or endoplasmic reticulum synthesize proteins after the process of transcription of DNA to RNA in the cell's nucleus. The entire process is called gene expression.

In translation, messenger RNA (mRNA) is decoded in a ribosome, outside the nucleus, to produce a specific amino acid chain, or polypeptide. The polypeptide later folds into an active protein and performs its functions in the cell. The ribosome facilitates decoding by inducing the binding of complementary tRNA anticodon sequences to mRNA codons. The tRNAs carry specific amino acids that are chained together into a polypeptide as the mRNA passes through and is "read" by the ribosome.

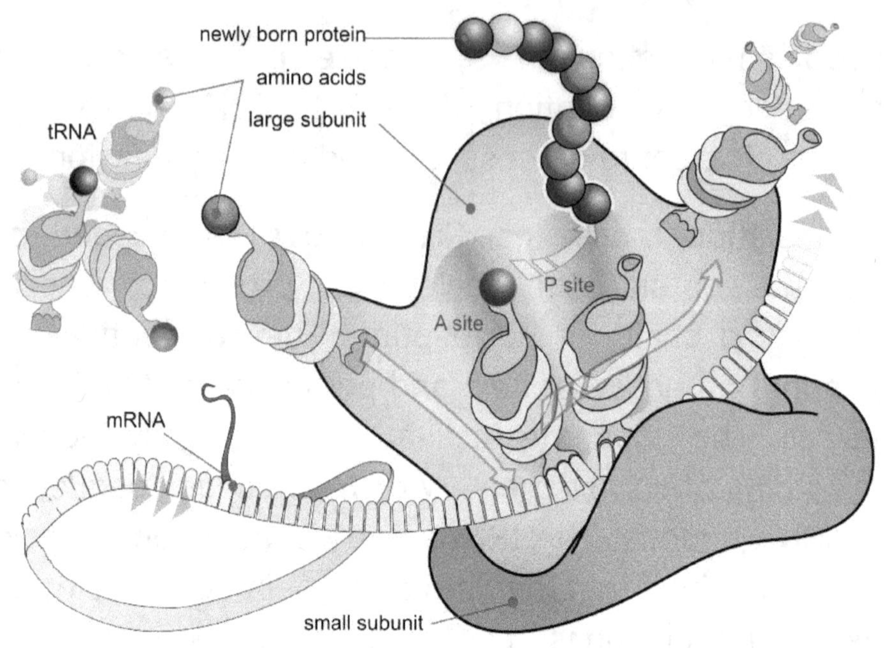



## Translation proceeds in three phases:

- **Initiation:** The ribosome assembles around the target mRNA. The first tRNA is attached at the start codon.

- **Elongation:** The last tRNA validated by the small ribosomal subunit (accommodation) transfers the amino acid it carries to the large ribosomal subunit which binds it to the one of the precedingly admitted tRNA (transpeptidation). The ribosome then moves to the next mRNA codon to continue the process (translocation), creating an amino acid chain.

- **Termination:** When a stop codon is reached, the ribosome releases the polypeptide. The ribosomal complex remains intact and moves on to the next mRNA to be translated.

In prokaryotes (bacteria and archaea), translation occurs in the cytosol, where the large and small subunits of the ribosome bind to the mRNA. In eukaryotes, translation occurs in the cytoplasm or across the membrane of the endoplasmic reticulum in a process called co-translational translocation. In co-translational translocation, the entire ribosome/mRNA complex binds to the outer membrane of the rough endoplasmic reticulum (ER) and the new protein is synthesized and released into the ER; the newly created polypeptide can be stored inside the ER for future vesicle transport and secretion outside the cell, or immediately secreted.

Many types of transcribed RNA, such as transfer RNA, ribosomal RNA, and small nuclear RNA, do not undergo translation into proteins.

A number of antibiotics act by inhibiting translation. These include anisomycin, cycloheximide, chloramphenicol, tetracycline, streptomycin, erythromycin, and puromycin. Prokaryotic ribosomes have a different structure from that of eukaryotic ribosomes, and thus antibiotics can specifically target bacterial infections without any harm to a eukaryotic host's cells.

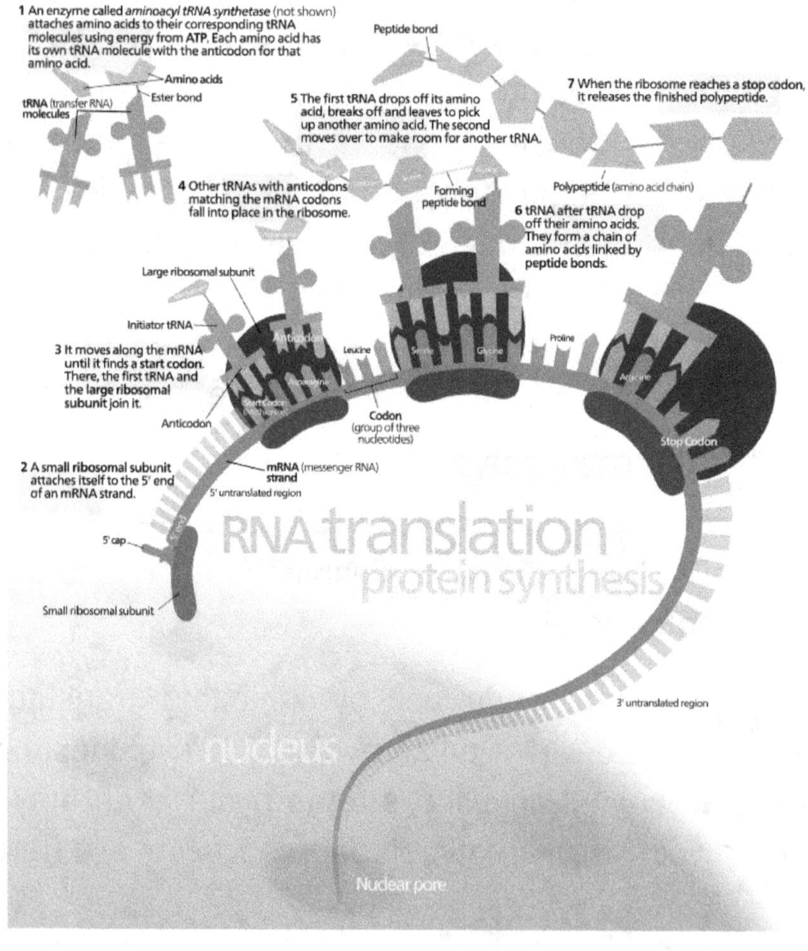

Small interfering RNA (siRNA), sometimes known as short interfering RNA or silencing RNA, is a class of double-stranded RNA at first non-coding RNA molecules, typically 20-24 (normally 21) base pairs in length, similar to miRNA, and operating within the RNA interference (RNAi) pathway. It interferes with the expression of specific genes with complementary nucleotide sequences by degrading mRNA after transcription, preventing translation

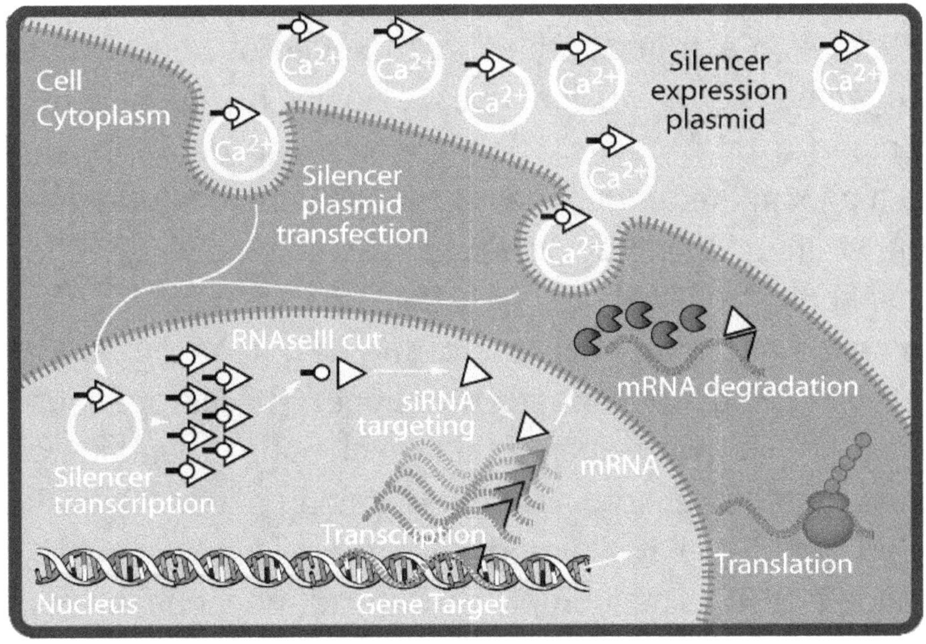


Deoxyribonucleic acid (listen); DNA) is a polymer composed of two polynucleotide chains that coil around

each other to form a double helix. The polymer carries genetic instructions for the development, functioning, growth and reproduction of all known organisms and many viruses. DNA and ribonucleic acid (RNA) are nucleic acids. Alongside proteins, lipids and complex carbohydrates (polysaccharides), nucleic acids are one of the four major types of macromolecules that are essential for all known forms of life.

The two DNA strands are known as polynucleotides as they are composed of simpler monomeric units called nucleotides Each nucleotide is composed of one of four nitrogen-containing nucleobases (cytosine [C], guanine [G], adenine [A] or thymine [T]), a sugar called deoxyribose, and a phosphate group. The nucleotides are joined to one another in a chain by covalent bonds (known as the phosphodiester linkage) between the sugar of one nucleotide and the phosphate of the next, resulting in an alternating sugar-phosphate backbone. The nitrogenous bases of the two separate polynucleotide strands are bound together, according to base pairing rules (A with T and C with G), with hydrogen bonds to make double-stranded DNA. The complementary nitrogenous bases are divided into two groups, pyrimidines and purines. In DNA, the pyrimidines are thymine and cytosine; the purines are adenine and guanine.

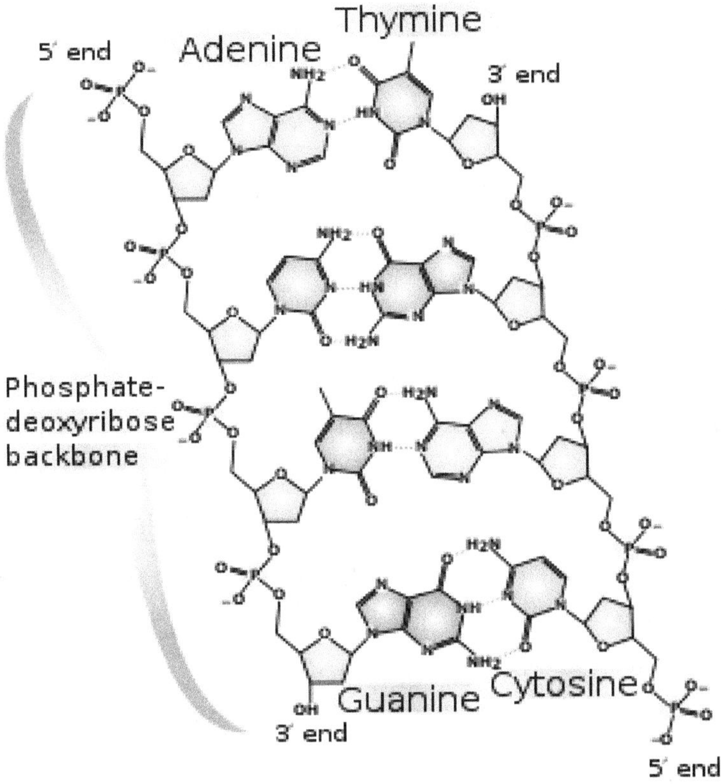

Both strands of double-stranded DNA store the same biological information. This information is replicated when the two strands separate. A large part of DNA (more than 98% for humans) is non-coding, meaning that these sections do not serve as patterns for protein sequences. The two strands of DNA run in opposite directions to each other and are thus antiparallel. Attached to each sugar is one of four types of nucleobases (or bases). It is the sequence of these four nucleobases along the backbone that encodes genetic information. RNA strands are created using DNA strands as a template in a process called transcription, where DNA bases are exchanged for their corresponding bases except in the case of thymine (T), for which RNA substitutes uracil (U).[4] Under the genetic code, these RNA strands specify the sequence of amino acids within proteins in a process called translation.

Within eukaryotic cells, DNA is organized into long structures called chromosomes. Before typical cell division, these chromosomes are duplicated in the process of DNA replication, providing a complete set of chromosomes for each daughter cell. Eukaryotic organisms (animals, plants, fungi and protists) store most of their DNA inside the cell nucleus as nuclear DNA, and some in the mitochondria as mitochondrial DNA or in chloroplasts as chloroplast DNA.[5] In contrast, prokaryotes (bacteria and archaea) store their DNA only in the cytoplasm, in circular chromosomes. Within eukaryotic chromosomes, chromatin proteins, such as histones, compact and organize DNA. These compacting structures guide the interactions between DNA and other proteins, helping control which parts of the DNA are transcribed.

# CHAPTER THREE

Epigenetics and Development

Developmental origins of health and disease

Epigenetics and stem cells

Trans generational epigenetics

- **Epigenetics and Development**

Epigenetics refers to the study of heritable changes in gene function that occur without a change in the underlying DNA sequence. These changes include modifications to the DNA molecule itself or to the proteins with which DNA interacts, such as histones. These modifications can affect how genes are expressed, which in turn can influence development.

During development, cells differentiate and specialize to form the various tissues and organs of an organism. Epigenetic mechanisms play a critical role in regulating gene expression during this process, allowing cells to respond to different signals and environments as they differentiate.

For example, the process of cell differentiation is often accompanied by changes in the pattern of histone modifications, which can cause certain genes to be repressed or activated. Additionally, microRNAs (ncRNAs) can also play important roles in the regulation of gene expression during development.

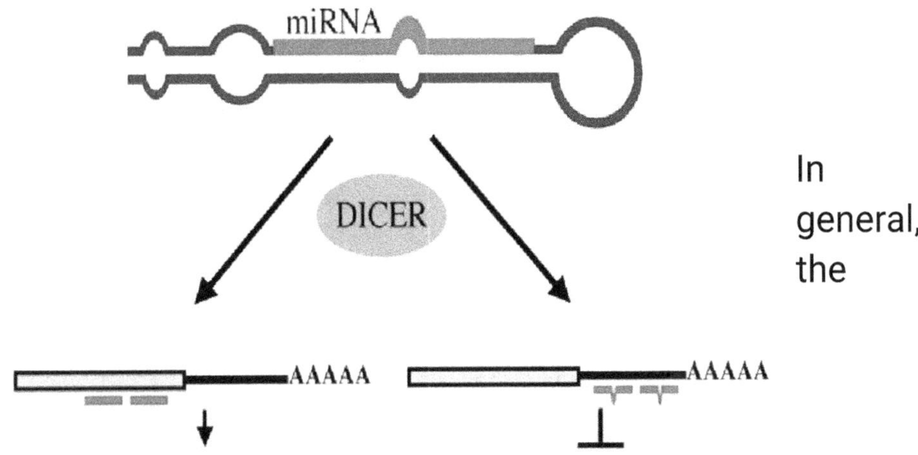



In general, the epigenetic modifications that occur during development are thought to help ensure that cells respond appropriately to the signals they receive and differentiate into the correct cell types. However, this process can also go wrong, leading to developmental disorders or diseases.

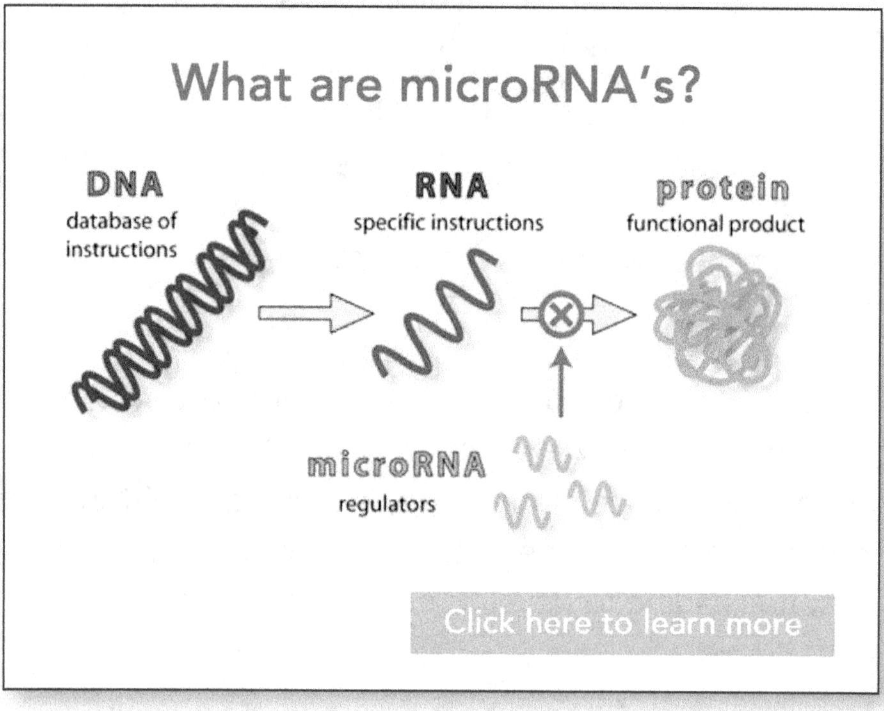

What are microRNA's?
DNA
database of
instructions
RNA
specific instructions
protein
functional product
microRNA
regulators
Click here to learn more

In traditional Chinese and other Asian cultures the aged were highly respected and cared for. The Igbo tribesmen of Eastern Nigeria value dependency in their aged and involve them in care of children and the administration of tribal affairs (Shelton, A. in Kalish R. Uni Michigan 1969).

In Eskimo culture the grandmother was pushed out into the ice-flow to die as soon as she became useless.

Western societies today usually resemble to some degree the Eskimo culture, only the "ice-flows" have names such a "Sunset Vista" and the like. Younger generations no longer assign status to the aged and their abandonment

is always in danger of becoming the social norm.

There has been a tendency to remove the aged from their homes and put them  in custodial care. To some degree the government provides domiciliary care services to prevent or delay this, but the motivation probably has more

to do with expense than humanity.

In Canada and some parts of the USA old people are being utilized as foster-grandparents in child care agencies.

## SOME BASIC DEFINITIONS

## What is Aging?

Aging: Aging is a natural phenomenon that refers to changes occurring throughout the life span and result in differences in structure and function between the youthful and elder generation.

Gerontology: Gerontology is the study of aging and includes science, psychology and sociology.

Geriatrics: A relatively new field of medicine specializing in the health problems of advanced age.

Social aging: Refers to the social habits and roles of individuals with respect to their culture and society. As social aging increases individual usually experience a decrease in meaningful social interactions.

Biological aging: Refers to the physical changes in the body systems during the later decades of life. It may begin long before the individual reaches chronological age 65.

Cognitive aging: Refers to decreasing ability to assimilate new information and learn new behaviours and skills.

## GENERAL PROBLEMS OF AGING

Eric Erikson (Youth and the life cycle. Children. 7:43-49 Mch/April 1960) developed an "ages and stages" theory of human development that involved 8 stages after birth each of which involved a basic dichotomy representing best case and worst case outcomes. Below are the dichotomies and their developmental relevance:

**Prenatal stage - conception to birth.**

1. Infancy. Birth to 2 years - basic trust vs. basic distrust. Hope.

2. Early childhood, 3 to 4 years - autonomy vs. self doubt/shame. Will.

3. Play age, 5 to 8 years - initiative vs. guilt. Purpose.

4. School age, 9to 12 - industry vs. inferiority. Competence.

5. Adolescence, 13 to 19 - identity vs. identity confusion. Fidelity.

6. Young adulthood - intimacy vs. isolation. Love.

7. Adulthood, generativity vs. self absorption. Care.

8. Mature age- Ego Integrity vs. Despair. Wisdom.

This stage of older adulthood, i.e. stage 8, begins about the time of retirement and continues throughout one's life. Achieving ego integrity  is a sign of maturity while failing to reach this stage is an indication of poor development in prior stages through the life course.

Ego integrity: This means coming to accept one's whole life and reflecting on it in a positive manner. According to Erikson, achieving integrity means fully accepting one' self and coming to terms with death. Accepting responsibility for one's life and being able to review the past with satisfaction is essential. The inability to do this leads to despair and the individual will begin to fear death. If a favorable balance is achieved during this stage, then wisdom is developed.

## Psychological and personality aspects:

Aging has psychological implications. Next to dying our recognition that we are aging may be one of the most profound shocks we ever receive. Once we pass the invisible line of 65 our years are bench marked for the remainder of the game of life. We are no longer "mature age" we are instead classified as "old", or "senior citizens". How we cope with the changes we face and stresses of altered status depends on our basic personality. Here are 3 basic personality types that have been identified. It may be a oversimplification but it makes the point about personality effectively:

    **a.** The autonomous - people who seem to have the resources for self-renewal. They may be dedicated to a goal or idea and committed to continuing productivity. This appears to protect them somewhat even against physiological aging.

**b.** The adjusted - people who are rigid and lacking in adaptability but are supported by their power, prestige or well structured routine. But if their situation changes drastically they become psychiatric casualties.

**c.** The anomic. These are people who do not have clear inner values or a protective life vision. Such people have been described as prematurely resigned and they may deteriorate rapidly.

## Summary of stresses of old age.

**a.** Retirement and reduced income. Most people rely on work for self worth, identity and social interaction. Forced retirement can be demoralising.

**b.** Fear of invalidism and death. The increased probability of falling prey to illness from which there is no recovery is a continual source of anxiety. When one has a heart attack or stroke the stress becomes much worse.

Some persons face death with equanimity, often psychologically supported by a religion or philosophy. Others may welcome death as an end to suffering or insoluble problems and with little concern for life or human existence. Still others face impending death with suffering of great stress against which they have no ego defenses.

**c.** Isolation and loneliness. Older people face inevitable loss of loved ones, friends and contemporaries. The loss of a spouse whom one has depended on for companionship and moral support is particularly distressing. Children grow up, marry and become preoccupied or move away. Failing memory, visual and aural impairment may all work to make social interaction difficult. And if this then leads to a souring of outlook and rigidity of attitude then social interaction becomes further lessened and the individual may not even utilize the avenues for social activity that are still available.

**d.** Reduction in sexual function and physical attractiveness. Kinsey et al, in their Sexual behavior in the human male,

(Phil., Saunders, 1948) found that there is a gradual decrease in sexual activity with advancing age and that reasonably gratifying patterns of sexual activity can continue into extreme old age. The aging person also has to adapt to loss of sexual attractiveness in a society which puts extreme emphasis on sexual attractiveness. The adjustment in self image and self concept that are required can be very hard to make.

**e**. Forces tending to self devaluation. Often the experience of the older generation has little perceived relevance to the problems of the young and the older person becomes deprived of participation in decision making both in occupational and family settings. Many parents are seen as unwanted burdens and their children may secretly wish they would die so they can be free of the burden and experience some financial relief or benefit. Senior citizens may be pushed into the role of being an old person with all this implies in terms of self devaluation.

## 4 Major Categories of Problems or Needs:

- Health.

- Housing.

- Income maintenance.

- Interpersonal relations.

## BIOLOGICAL CHANGES

Physiological Changes: Catabolism (the breakdown of protoplasm) overtakes anabolism (the build-up of protoplasm). All body systems are affected and repair systems become slowed. The aging process occurs at different rates in different individuals.

**Physical appearance and other changes:**

Loss of subcutaneous fat and less elastic skin gives rise to wrinkled appearance, sagging and loss of smoothness of body contours. Joints stiffen and become painful and range of joint movement becomes restricted, general

mobility lessened.

## Respiratory changes:

Increase of fibrous tissue in chest walls and lungs leads restricts respiratory movement and less oxygen is consumed. Older people more likelyto have lower respiratory infections whereas young people have upper respiratory infections.

## Nutritive changes:

Tooth decay and loss of teeth can detract from ease and enjoyment in eating. Atrophy of the taste buds means food is inclined to be tasteless and this should be taken into account by careers. Digestive changes occur from lack of exercise (stimulating intestines) and decrease in digestive juice production. Constipation and indigestion are likely to follow as a result. Financial problems can lead to the elderly eating an excess of cheap carbohydrates rather than the more expensive protein and vegetable foods and this exacerbates the problem, leading to reduced vitamin intake and such problems as anemia and increased susceptibility to infection.

## Adaptation to stress:

All of us face stress at all ages. Adaptation to stress requires the consumption of energy. The 3 main phases of stress are:

**1. Initial alarm reaction. 2. Resistance. 3. Exhaustion**

and if stress continues tissue damage or aging occurs. Older persons have had a lifetime of dealing with stresses. Energy reserves are depleted and the older person succumbs to stress earlier than the younger person. Stress is cumulative over a lifetime. Research results, including experiments with animals suggests that each stress leaves us more vulnerable to the next and that although we might think we've "bounced back" 100% in fact each stress leaves it scar. Further, stress is psycho-biological meaning

the kind of stress is irrelevant. A physical stress may leave one more vulnerable to psychological stress and vice versa. Rest does not completely restore one after a stressor. Care workers need to be mindful of this and cognizant of the kinds of things that can produce stress for aged persons.

**COGNITIVE CHANGE** Habitual Behavior:

Sigmund Freud noted that after the age of 50, treatment of neuroses via psychoanalysis was difficult because the opinions and reactions of older people were relatively fixed and hard to shift.

Over-learned behavior: This is behavior that has been learned so well and repeated so often that it has become automatic, like for example typing or running down stairs. Over-learned behavior is hard to change. If one has lived a long time one is likely to have fixed opinions and ritualized behavior patterns or habits.

Compulsive behavior: Habits and attitudes that have been learned in the course of finding ways to overcome frustration and difficulty are very hard to break. Tension reducing habits such as nail biting, incessant humming, smoking or drinking alcohol are especially hard to change at any age and particularly hard for persons who have been practicing them over a life time.

The psychology of over-learned and compulsive behaviours has severe implications for older persons who find they have to live in what for them is a new and alien environment with new rules and power relations.

**Information acquisition:**

Older people have a continual background of neural noise making it more difficult for them to sort out and interpret complex sensory

input. In talking to an older person one should turn off the TV, eliminate as many noises and distractions as possible, talk slowly and relate to one message or idea at a time.

Memories from the distant past are stronger than more

recent memories. New memories are the first to fade and last to return.

Time patterns also can get mixed - old and new may get mixed.

**Intelligence.**

Intelligence reaches a peak and can stay high with little deterioration if there is no neurological damage. People who have unusually high intelligence to begin with seem to suffer the least decline. Education and stimulation also seem to play a role in maintaining intelligence.

Intellectual impairment. Two diseases of old age causing cognitive decline are Alzheimer's syndrome and Pick's syndrome. In Pick's syndrome there is inability to concentrate and learn and also affective responses are impaired.

Degenerative Diseases: Slow progressive physical degeneration of cells in the nervous system. Genetics appear to be an important factor. Usually start after age 40 (but can occur as early as 20s).

**ALZHEIMER'S DISEASE** Degeneration of all areas of cortex but particularly frontal and temporal lobes. The affected cells actually die. Early symptoms resemble neurotic disorders: Anxiety, depression, restlessness sleep difficulties.

Progressive deterioration of all intellectual faculties (memory deficiency being the most well known and obvious). Total mass of the brain decreases, ventricles become larger. No established treatment.

**PICK'S DISEASE** Rare degenerative disease. Similar to Alzheimer's in terms of onset, symptomatology and possible genetic etiology. However it affects circumscribed areas of the brain, particularly the frontal areas which leads to a loss of normal affect.

**PARKINSON'S DISEASE** Neuropathology: Loss of neurons in the basal ganglia.

Symptoms: Movement abnormalities: rhythmical alternating tremor of extremities, eyelids and tongue along with rigidity of the muscles and slowness of movement (akinesia).

It was once thought that Parkinson's disease was not associated with intellectual deterioration, but it is now known that there is an association between global intellectual impairment and Parkinson's where it occurs late in life.

The cells lost in Parkinson's are associated with the neuro -chemical Dopamine and the motor symptoms of

Parkinson's are associated the dopamine deficiency. Treatment involves administration of dopamine precursor L-dopa which can alleviate symptoms including intellectual impairment. Research suggests it may possibly bring to the fore emotional effects in patients who have had psychiatric illness at some prior stage in their lives.

**AFFECTIVE DOMAIN** In old age our self concept gets its final revision. We make a final assessment of the value of our lives and our balance of success and failures.

How well a person adapts to old age may be predicated by how well the person adapted to earlier significant changes. If the person suffered an emotional crisis each time a significant change was needed then adaptation to the exigencies of old age may also be difficult. Factors such as economic security, geographic location and physical health are important to the adaptive process.

**Need Fulfillment:** For all of us, according to Maslow's Hierarchy of Needs theory, we are not free to pursue the higher needs of self actualization unless the basic needs are secured. When one considers that many, perhaps most, old people are living in poverty and continually concerned with basic survival needs, they are not likely to be happily satisfying needs related to prestige, achievement and beauty.

Maslow's Hierarchy

Physiological

Safety

Belonging, love, identification

Esteem: Achievement, prestige, success, self respect

Self actualization: Expressing one's interests and talents to the full.

Note: Old people who have secured their basic needs may be motivated to work on tasks of the highest levels in the hierarchy - activities concerned with aesthetics, creativity and altruistic matters, as compensation for loss of sexual attractiveness and athleticism. Aged care workers fixated on getting old people to focus on social activities may only succeed in frustrating and irritating them if their basic survival concerns are not secured to their satisfaction.

## DISENGAGEMENT

Social aging according to Cumming, E. and Henry, W. (Growing old: the aging process of disengagement, NY, Basic 1961) follows a well defined pattern:

1. Change in role. Change in occupation and productivity. Possibly change

in attitude to work.

2. Loss of role, e.g. retirement or death of a husband.

3. Reduced social interaction. With loss of role social interactions are

diminished, eccentric adjustment can further reduce social interaction, damage

to self concept, depression.

4. Awareness of scarcity of remaining time. This produces further curtailment of

activity in interest of saving time.

Havighurst, R. et al (in B. Negatron (ed.) Middle age and aging, U. of Chicago, 1968) and others have suggested that disengagement is not an inevitable process. They believe the needs of the old are essentially the same as in middle age and the activities of middle age should be extended as long as possible. Havighurst points out the decrease in social interaction of the aged is often largely the result of society withdrawing from the individual as much as the reverse. To combat this he believes the individual must vigorously resist the limitations of his social world.

**DEATH** The fear of the dead amongst tribal societies is

well established. Persons who had ministered to the dead were taboo and required observe various rituals including seclusion for varying periods of time. In some societies from South America to Australia it is taboo for certain persons to utter the name of the dead. Widows and widowers are expected to observe rituals in respect for the dead.

Widows in the Highlands of New Guinea around Goroka chop of one of their own fingers. The dead continue their existence as spirits and upsetting them can bring dire consequences.

Wahl, C in "The fear of death", 1959 noted that the fear of death occurs as early as the 3rd year of life. When a child loses a pet or grandparent fears reside in the unspoken questions: Did I cause it? Will happen to you (parent) soon? Will this happen to me? The child in such situations needs to re-assure that the departure is not a censure, and that the parent is not likely to depart soon. Love, grief, guilt, anger are a mix of conflicting emotions that are experienced.

## CONTEMPORARY ATTITUDES TO DEATH

Our culture places high value on youth, beauty, high status occupations, social class and anticipated future activities and achievement. Aging and dying are denied and avoided in this system. The death of each person reminds us of our own mortality.

The death of the elderly is less disturbing to members of Western society because the aged are not especially valued. Surveys have established that nurses for example attach more importance to saving a young life than an old life. In Western society there is a pattern of avoiding dealing with the aged and dying aged patient.

Stages of dying. Elisabeth Kubler Ross has specialized in working with dying patients and in her "On death and dying", NY, Macmillan, 1969, summarized 5 stages in dying.

1. Denial and isolation. "No, not me".

2. Anger. "I've lived a good life so why me?"

3. Bargaining. Secret deals are struck with God. "If I can live until...I promise to..."

4. Depression. (In general the greatest psychological problem of the aged is depression). Depression results from real and threatened loss.

## 5. Acceptance of the inevitable.

Kubler Ross's typology as set out above should, I believe be taken with a grain of salt and not slavishly accepted.

Celebrated US Journalist David Rieff who was in June '08 a guest of the Sydney writer's festival in relation to his book, "Swimming in a sea of death: a son's memoir" (Melbourne University Press) expressly denied the validity of the Kubler Ross typology in his Late Night Live interview (Australian ABC radio) with Philip Adams June 9th '08. He said something to the effect that his mother had regarded her impending death as murder. My own experience with dying persons suggests that the human ego is extraordinarily resilient. I recall visiting a dying colleague in hospital just days before his death. He said, "I'm dying, I don't like it but there's nothing I can do about it", and then went on to chortle about how senior academics at an Adelaide university had told him they were submitting his name for a the Order of Australia (the new "Knighthood" replacement in Australia). Falling in and out of lucid thought with an oxygen tube in his nostrils he was nevertheless still highly interested in the "vain glories of the world". This observation to me seemed consistent with Rieff's negative assessment of Kubler Ross's theories.


## THE AGED IN RELATION TO YOUNGER PEOPLE

The aged share with the young the same needs: However, the aged often have fewer or weaker resources to meet those needs. Their need for social interaction may be ignored by family and care workers.

Family should make time to visit their aged members and invite them to their homes. The aged like to visit children and relate to them through games and stories.

Meaningful relationships can be developed via foster-grandparent programs. Some aged are not aware of their income and health entitlements. Family and friends should take the time to explain these. Some aged are too proud to access their entitlements and this problem should be addressed in a kindly way where it occurs.

It is best that the aged be allowed as much choice as possible in matters related to living arrangements, social life and lifestyle.

Communities serving the aged need to provide for the aged via such things as lower curbing, and ramps.

Careers need to examine their own attitude to aging and dying. Denial in the carer is detected by the aged person and it can inhibit the aged person from expressing negative feelings - fear, anger. If the person can express these feelings to someone then that person is less likely to die with a sense of isolation and bitterness.

# A METAPHYSICAL PERSPECTIVE

The following notes are my interpretation of a Dr. Depak Chopra lecture entitled, "The New Physics of Healing" which he presented to the 13th Scientific Conference of the American Holistic Medical Association. Dr. Depak Chopra is an endocrinologist and a former Chief of Staff of New England Hospital, Massachusetts. I am deliberately omitting the detail of his explanations of the more abstract, ephemeral and controversial ideas.

In the lecture Dr. Chopra presents a model of the universe and of all organisms as structures of interacting centers of electromagnetic energy linked to each other in such a way that anything affecting one part of a system or structure has ramifications throughout the entire structure. This model becomes an analogue not only for what happens within the structure or organism itself, but between the organism and both its physical and social environments. In other words there is a correlation between psychological conditions, health and the aging process. Dr. Chopra in his lecture reconciles ancient Vedic (Hindu) philosophy with modern psychology and quantum physics.

Premature Precognitive Commitment: Dr. Chopra invokes experiments that have shown that flies kept for a long time in a jar do not quickly leave the jar when the top is taken off. Instead they accept the jar as the limit of their universe. He also points out that in India baby elephants are often kept tethered to a small twig or sapling. In adulthood when the elephant is capable of pulling over a medium sized tree it can still be successfully tethered to a twig! As another example he points to experiments in which fish are bred on 2 sides of a fish tank containing a divider between the 2 sides. When the divider is removed the fish are slow to learn that they can now swim throughout the whole tank but rather stay in the section that they accept as their universe. Other experiments have demonstrated that kittens brought up in an environment of vertical stripes and structures, when released in adulthood keep bumping into anything aligned horizontally as if they were unable to see anything that is horizontal. Conversely kittens brought up in an environment of horizontal stripes when released bump into vertical structures, apparently unable to see them.

The whole point of the above experiments is that they demonstrate Premature Precognitive Commitment. The lesson to be learned is that our sensory apparatus develops as a result of initial experience and how we've been taught to interpret it.

What is the real look of the world? It doesn't exist. The way the world looks to us is determined by the sensory receptors we have and our interpretation of that look is determined by our premature precognitive commitments. Dr Chopra makes the point that less than a billionth of the available stimuli make it into our nervous systems. Most of it is screened, and what gets through to us is whatever we are expecting to find on the basis of our precognitive commitments.

Dr. Chopra also discusses the diseases that are actually caused by mainstream medical interventions, but this material gets too far away from my central intention. Dr. Chopra discusses in lay terms the physics of matter, energy and time by way of establishing the wider context of our existence. He makes the point that our bodies including the bodies of plants are mirrors of cosmic rhythms and exhibit changes correlating even with the tides.

Dr. Chopra cites the experiments of Dr. Herbert Spencer of the US National Institute of Health. He injected mice with Poly-IC, an immune-stimulant while making the mice repeatedly smell camphor. After the effect of the Poly-IC had worn off he again exposed the mice to the camphor smell. The smell of camphor had the effect of causing the mice's immune system to automatically strengthen

as if they had been injected with the stimulant. He then took another batch of mice and injected them with cyclophosphamide which tends to destroy the immune system while exposing them to the smell of camphor. Later after being returned to normal just the smell of camphor was enough to cause destruction of their immune system. Dr. Chopra points out that whether or not camphor enhanced or destroyed the mice's immune system was entirely determined by an interpretation of the meaning of the smell of camphor. The interpretation is not just in the brain but in each cell of the organism. We are bound to our imagination and our Early experiences.

Chopra cites a study by the Massachusetts Dept of Health Education and Welfare into risk factors for heart disease - family history, cholesterol etc. The 2 most important risk factors were found to be psychological measures - Self Happiness Rating and Job Satisfaction. They found most people died of heart disease on a Monday!

Chopra says that for every feeling there is a molecule. If you are experiencing tranquillity your body will be producing natural valium. Chemical changes in the brain are reflected by changes in other cells including blood cells. The brain produces neuropeptides and brain structures are chemically tuned to these neuropeptide receptors. Neuropeptides (neurotransmitters) are the chemical concommitants of thought. Chopra points out the white blood cells (a part of the immune system) have neuropeptide receptors and are "eavesdropping" on our thinking. Conversely the immune system produces its own neuropeptides which can influence the nervous system. He goes on to say that cells in all parts of the body including heart and kidneys for example also produce neuropeptides and neuopeptide sensitivity. Chopra assures us that most neurologists would agree that the nervous system and the immune system are parallel systems.

Other studies in physiology: The blood interlukin-2 levels of medical students decreased as exam time neared and their interlukin receptor capacities also lowered. Chopra says if we are having fun to the point of exhilaration our natural interlukin-2 levels become higher. Interlukin-2 is a powerful and very expensive anti-cancer drug. The body is a printout of consciousness. If we could change the way we look at our bodies at a genuine, profound level then our bodies would actually change.

On the subject of "time" Chopra cites Sir Thomas Gall and Steven Hawkins, stating that our description of the universe as having a past, present, and future are constructed entirely out of our interpretation of change. But in reality linear time doesn't exist.

Chopra explains the work of Alexander Leaf a former

Harvard Professor of Preventative Medicine who toured the world investigating societies where people lived beyond 100 years (these included parts of Afghanistan, Soviet Georgia, Southern Andes). He looked at possible factors including climate, genetics, and diet. Leaf concluded the most important factor was the collective perception of aging in these societies.

Amongst the Tama Humana of the Southern Andes there was a collective belief that the older you got the more physically able you got. They had a tradition of running and the older one became then generally the better at running one got. The best runner was aged 60. Lung capacity and other measures actually improved with age. People were healthy until well into their 100s and died in their sleep. Chopra remarks that things have changed since the introduction of Budweiser (beer) and TV.

[DISCUSSION: How might TV be a factor in changing the former ideal state of things?]

Chopra refers to Dr. Ellen Langor a former Harvard Psychology professor's work. Langor advertised for 100 volunteers aged over 70 years. She took them to a Monastery outside Boston to play "Let's Pretend". They were divided into 2 groups each of which resided in a different part of the building. One group, the control group spent several days talking about the 1950s. The other group, the experimental group had to live as if in the year 1959 and talk about it in the present tense. What appeared on their TV screens were the old newscasts and movies. They read old newspapers and magazines of the period. After 3 days everyone was photographed and the photographs judged by independent judges who knew nothing of the nature of the experiment. The experimental group seemed to have gotten younger in appearance. Langor then arranged for them to be tested for 100 physiological parameters of aging which included of course blood pressure, near point vision and DHEA levels. After 10 days of living as if in 1959 all parameters had reversed by the equivalent of at least 20 years.

Chopra concludes from Langor's experiment: "We are the metabolic end product of our sensory experiences. How we interpret them depends on the collective mindset which influences individual biological entropy and aging."

Can one escape the current collective mindset and reap the benefits in longevity and health? Langor says, society won't let you escape. There are too many reminders of how most people think linear time is and how it expresses itself in entropy and aging - men are naughty at 40 and on social welfare at 55, women reach menopause at 40 etc. We get to see so many other people aging and dying that it sets the pattern that we follow.

Chopra concludes we are the metabolic product of our sensory experience and our interpretation gets structured in our biology itself. Real change comes from change in the collective consciousness - otherwise it cannot occur within the individual.

## • Epigenetics and stem cells

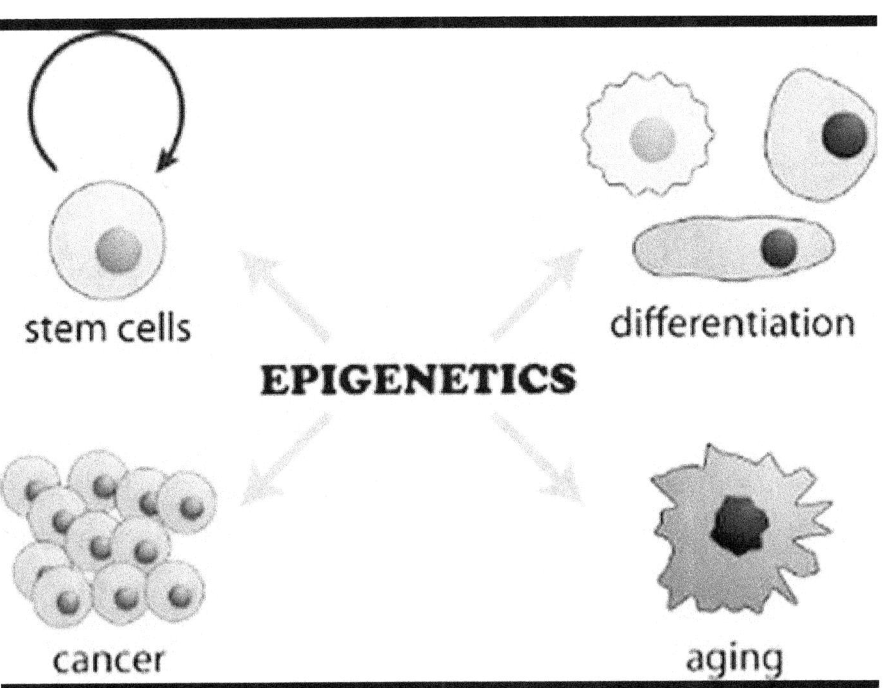


stem cells
differentiation
EPIGENETICS
cancer
aging


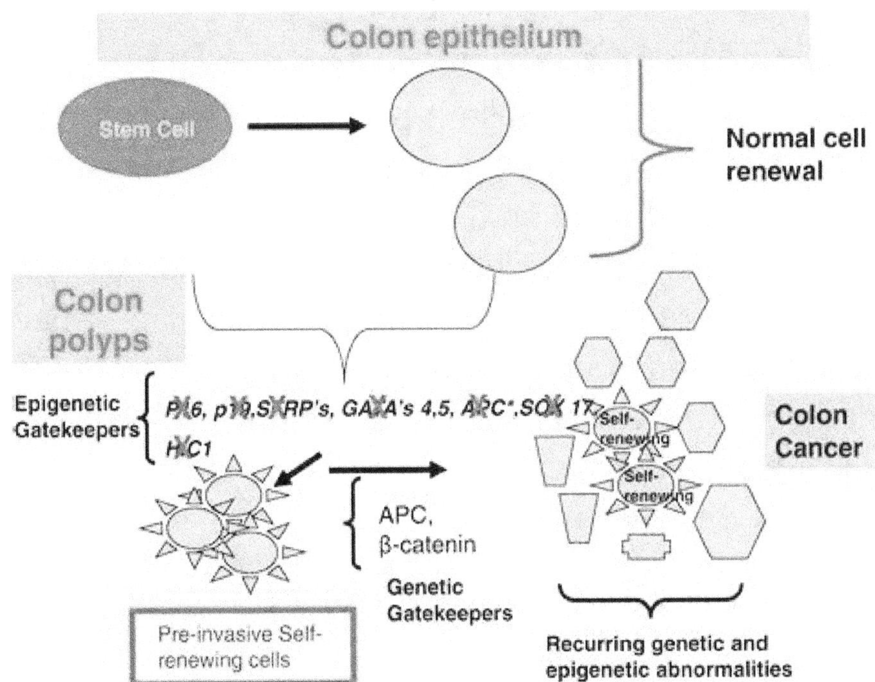


Colon epithelium
Stem Cell
Normal cell renewal
Colon polyps
Epigenetic Gatekeepers
P16, p19, SFRP's, GATA's 4,5, APC, SOX 17, HIC1
APC, β-catenin
Genetic Gatekeepers
Pre-invasive Self-renewing cells
Self-renewing
Self-renewing
Colon Cancer
Recurring genetic and epigenetic abnormalities

Epigenetics is the study of heritable changes in gene function that do not involve changes to the underlying DNA sequence. These changes can include modifications to the DNA molecule itself or to the proteins with which DNA interacts. One of the most well-known epigenetic modifications is DNA methylation, which involves the addition of a methyl group to the DNA molecule.

Stem cells are a special type of cell that have the ability to differentiate into many different cell types. They also have the ability to self-renew, meaning they can divide and produce more stem cells. There are two main types of stem cells: embryonic stem cells, which are derived from early-stage embryos, and adult stem cells, which are found in various tissues throughout the body.

The field of epigenetic is particularly important in the study of stem cells because it plays a crucial role in the regulation of stem cell behavior. Epigenetic modifications can determine whether a stem cell remains in a dormant state or begins to differentiate into a specific cell type. For example, certain patterns of DNA methylation have been associated with the maintenance of stem cell pluripotency (the ability to differentiate into any cell type), while other patterns have been associated with the initiation of differentiation.

Epigenetic changes also play a role in stem cell aging and

reprogramming. As stem cells divide, they can accumulate mutations in their epigenetic marks which can cause them to lose their self-renewal and pluripotency properties. Reprogramming of somatic cells (non-stem cells) into induced pluripotent stem cells (iPSCs) is a way to reverse these epigenetic changes to generate a new population of pluripotent stem cells.

In summary, Epigenetics is the study of heritable changes in gene function and it plays a crucial role in the regulation of stem cell behavior, including maintenance of pluripotency, initiation of differentiation and stem cell aging and reprogramming.

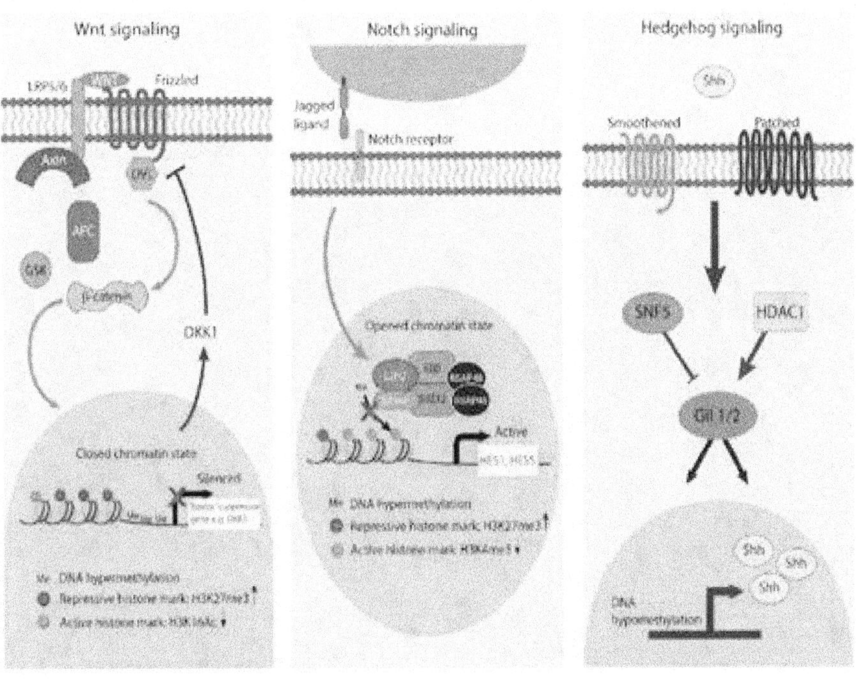

# • Tran's generational Epigenetics

Tran generational epigenetic inheritance, often known as epigenetically, is the transmission of epigenetic markers from one organism to the next (i.e., from parent to kid) that alters the phenotypes of offspring without changing the DNA's fundamental structure (i.e., the nucleotide sequence) Information transfer between cells and between organisms may be covered under the less exact phrase "epigenetic inheritance." Nevertheless, these two levels of epigenetic.

While epigenetic inheritance is same in unicellular species, multicellular organisms may have different processes and evolutionary differences.

Some people believe that because of epigenetic, modern biology no longer strongly opposes the inheritance of acquired characteristics (Lamarckism), as it once did. Environmental factors can induce the epigenetic marks (epigenetic tags) for some epigenetically influenced traits, whereas some marks are heritable.

**There are four main types of epigenetic modification:**

Prions, proteins that replicate by altering the structure of normal proteins to match their own, structural templating, in which structures are replicated using a template or scaffold structure on the parent, the orientation and architecture of cytoskeleton structures, cilia and flagella, and chromatin marks, in which mRNA or protein products of a gene stimulate transcription of the gene;

RNA silencing, in which small RNA strands interfere (RNAi) with the transcription of DNA or translation of mRNA; known only from a few studies, mostly in Caenorhabditis elegans

Even though there are many ways to inherit epigenetic markers, the process may be summed up as the transfer of epigenetic information along the germ line. Additionally, epigenetic variation normally manifests in one of four broad ways, while there may be additional, as-yet-unidentified forms. Individual cell epigenes are now altered through self-sustaining feedback loops, spatial templating, chromatin tagging, and RNA-mediated mechanisms. Either endogenous or external diversity in epigenetic patterns exists in multicellular organisms. Exogenous is a cellular reaction to environmental inputs, whereas endogenous is produced through cell-cell signaling (for instance, during early development when cells are differentiating).

# Removing versus keeping

Although some epigenetic reactions have been demonstrated to be conserved, such as transposon methylation in plants, a large portion of the epigenetic alteration within cells is reset after meiosis in sexually reproducing animals. The assignment of epigenetic causation to some parent of origin effects in animals and plants may result from differential inheritance of epigenetic marks caused by underlying maternal or paternal biases in removal or retention mechanisms.

# Reprogramming

Epigenetic alterations in animals occur twice during the course of the life cycle. Following fertilization, and then in the growing primordial germ cells, which are the forerunners of future gametes. The male and female gametes unite during fertilization in various cell cycle phases and with various genomic configurations. The male's epigenetic marks quickly disappear. The histones associated with the male DNA are first replaced with those from the female's cytoplasm, the majority of which are acetylated either because there are more acetylated histones in the female's cytoplasm or because the male

DNA preferentially binds to acetylated histones. Second, many species routinely demethylate the male DNA, potentially by means of 5-hydroxymethylcytosine.

Parental imprinting results when certain epigenetic markers, particularly maternal DNA methylation, manage to evade this reprogramming.

There is a more widespread deletion of epigenetic information in the primordial germ cells (PGC). However, some uncommon locations can also avoid DNA methylation erasure. [18] Epigenetic inheritance across generations may be possible if epigenetic marks manage to avoid being erased during both zygotic and PGC reprogramming events.

Recently, interest in manipulating epigenetic programming has increased due to the realization of how crucial it is to the establishment and fixation of cell line identity during early embryogenesis. [19] Regenerative medicine may become more widely used if epigenetic alterations enable the restoration of totipotency in stem cells or other types of cells.

## Retention

Some epigenetic marks may be co-transmitted via cellular systems. The DNA processivity factor proliferating cell nuclear antigen (PCNA), which has also been linked to patterning and strand crosstalk that enables copy fidelity of epigenetic marks, couples DNA polymerases acting on the leading and lagging strands during replication. Although research on histone modification copy fidelity is still in the model stage, preliminary findings indicate that new Histone modifications are modeled after those of the old histones and that new and old histones are distributed randomly across the two daughter DNA strands. In terms of transmission to the following generation,

numerous marks are eliminated as previously said. Patterns of epigenetic conservation across generations are being discovered by recent investigations. For instance, demethylation is resistant to centromeric satellites. Though the exact mechanism underlying this conservation is unknown, some data point to the possibility that histone methylation may play a role. There was additional evidence of promoter methylation timing dysregulation linked to embryonic gene expression dysregulation.

## Decay

Whereas the mutation rate in a given 100-base gene may be 10–7 per generation, epigenes may "mutate" several times per generation or may be fixed for many generations. This raises the question: do changes in epigene frequencies constitute evolution? Rapidly decaying epigenetic effects on phenotypes (i.e. lasting less than three generations) may explain some of the residual variation in phenotypes after genotype and environment are accounted for. However, distinguishing these short-term effects from the effects of the maternal environment on early ontogeny remains a challenge.

## Contribution to phenotypes

The relative importance of genetic and epigenetic inheritance is subject to debate though hundreds of examples of epigenetic modification of phenotypes have been published, few studies have been conducted outside of the laboratory setting. Therefore, the interactions of genes and epigenes with the environment cannot be inferred despite the central role of environment in natural selection. Experimental methodologies for manipulating epigenetic mechanisms are nascent and will need rigorous demonstration before studies explicitly testing the relative contributions of genotype, environment, and epigenotype are feasible.

## IN PLANTS

Studies concerning transgenerational epigenetic inheritance in plants have been reported as early as the 1950s. One of the earliest and best characterized examples of this is b1 paramutation in maize. The b1 gene encodes a basic helix-loop-helix transcription factor that is involved in the anthocyanin production pathway. When the b1 gene is expressed, the plant accumulates anthocyanin within its tissues, leading to a purple coloration of those tissues. The B-I allele (for B-Intense) has high expression of b1 resulting in the dark pigmentation of the sheath and husk tissues while the B' (pronounced B-prime) allele has low expression of b1 resulting in low pigmentation in those tissues. When homozygous B-I parents are crossed to homozygous B', the resultant F1 offspring all display low pigmentation which is due to gene silencing of b1. Unexpectedly, when F1 plants are self-crossed, the resultant F2 generation all display low pigmentation and have low levels of b1 expression. Furthermore, when any F2 plant (including those that are genetically homozygous for B-I) are crossed to homozygous B-I, the offspring will all display low pigmentation and expression of b1. The lack of darkly pigmented individuals in the F2 progeny is an example of non-Mendelian inheritance and further research has suggested that the B-I allele is converted to B' via epigenetic mechanisms. The B' and B-I alleles are considered to be epialleles because they are identical at the DNA sequence level but differ in the level of DNA methylation, siRNA production, and chromosomal interactions within the nucleus..  Additionally, plants defective in components of the RNA-directed DNA-methylation pathway show an increased expression of b1 in B' individuals similar to that of B-I, however, once these components are restored, the plant reverts to the low expression state. Although spontaneous conversion from B-I to B' has been observed, a reversion from B' to B-I (green to purple) has never been observed over 50 years and thousands of plants in both greenhouse and field experiments.

Examples of environmentally induced transgenerational epigenetic inheritance in plants has also been reported. In one case, rice plants that were exposed to drought-simulation treatments displayed increased tolerance to drought after 11 generations of exposure and propagation by single-seed descent as compared to non-drought treated plants. Differences in drought tolerance was linked to directional changes in DNA-methylation levels throughout the genome, suggesting that stress-induced heritable changes in DNA-methylation patterns may be important in adaptation to recurring stresses. In another study, plants that were exposed to moderate caterpillar herbivory over multiple generations displayed increased resistance to herbivory in subsequent generations (as measured by caterpillar dry mass) compared to plants lacking herbivore pressure.

This increase in herbivore resistance persisted after a generation of growth without any herbivore exposure suggesting that the response was transmitted across generations. The report concluded that components of the RNA-directed DNA-methylation pathway are involved in the increased resistance across generations. Transgenerational epigenetic inheritance has also been observed in polyploid plants. Genetically identical reciprocal F1 hybrid triploids have been shown to display transgenerational epigenetic effects on viable F2 seed development.

## In humans

Although genetic inheritance is important when describing phenotypic outcomes, it cannot entirely explain why offspring resemble their parents. Aside from genes, offspring come to inherit similar environmental conditions established by previous generations.

One environment that human offspring commonly share for nine months is the womb. Considering the duration of the fetal stages of development, the environment of the mother's womb can have long lasting effects on the health of offspring.[9]

An example of how the environment within the

womb can affect the health of an offspring is the Dutch hunger winter and its causal effect on induced transgenerational epigenetic inherited diseases.[9]

A number of studies suggest the existence of transgenerational epigenetic inheritance in humans, which includes the Dutch famine of 1944–45.

During the Dutch hunger winter, the offspring born during the famine were smaller than those born the year before the famine. The effects of this famine on development lasted up to two generations.

Moreover, the offspring born during the famine were found to have an increased risk of glucose intolerance in adulthood.

Differential DNA methylation has been found in adult female offspring who had been exposed to famine in utero, but it is unknown whether these differences in DNA methylation were passed on to their germ line.

It is hypothesized that inhibiting the PIM3 gene may have caused slower metabolism in later generations, but causation has not been proven, only correlation. The phenomenon is sometimes referred to as Dutch Hunger Winter Syndrome.

Furthermore, the increased rates of metabolic

diseases, cardiovascular diseases, and other increased risk factors to the health of F1 and F2 generations during the Dutch hunger winter is a known phenomenon called "fetal programming," which is caused by exposure to harmful environmental factors in utero.[9]

Another study hypothesized that epigenetic changes on the Y chromosome could explain differences in lifespan among the male descendants of prisoners of war in the American Civil War.


The Överkalix study noted sex-specific effects; a greater body mass index (BMI) at 9 years in sons, but not daughters, of fathers who began smoking early.

The paternal grandfather's food supply was only linked to the mortality RR of grandsons and not granddaughters. The paternal grandmother's food supply was only associated with the granddaughters' mortality risk ratio. When the grandmother had a good food supply was associated with a twofold higher mortality (RR).

This transgenerational inheritance was observed with exposure during the slow growth period (SGP). The SGP is the time before the start of puberty, when environmental factors have a larger impact on the body. The ancestors' SGP in this study was set between the ages of 9-12 for boys and 8–10 years for girls. This occurred in the SGP of both grandparents, or during the gestation period/infant life of the grandmothers, but not during either grandparent's puberty.

The father's poor food supply and the mother's good food supply were associated with a lower risk of cardiovascular death.

The loss of genetic expression which results in Prader–Willi syndrome or Angelman syndrome has in some cases been found to be caused by epigenetic changes (or "epimutations") on both the alleles, rather than involving any genetic mutation. In all 19 informative cases, the epimutations that, together with physiological imprinting and therefore silencing of the other allele, were causing these syndromes were localized on a chromosome with a specific parental and grandparental origin. Specifically, the paternally derived chromosome carried an abnormal maternal mark at the SNURF-SNRPN, and this abnormal mark was inherited from the paternal grandmother.

Similarly, epimutations on the MLH1 gene has been found in two individuals with a phenotype of hereditary nonpolyposis colorectal cancer, and without any frank MLH1 mutation which otherwise causes the disease. The same epimutations were also found on the spermatozoa of one of the individuals, indicating the potential to be transmitted to offspring.

In addition to epimutations to the MLH1 gene, it has been determined that certain cancers, such as breast cancer, can originate during the fetal stages within the uterus.

Furthermore, evidence collected in various studies utilizing model systems (i.e. animals) have found that exposure during parental generations can result in multigenerational and transgenerational inheritance of breast cancer.

More recently, studies have discovered a connection between the adaptation of male germinal cells via pre-conception paternal diets and the regulation of breast cancer in developing offspring. More specifically, studies have begun to uncover new data that underscores a relationship between transgenerational epigenetic inheritance of breast cancer and ancestral alimentary components or associated markers, such as birth weight.

By utilizing model systems, such as mice, studies have shown that stimulated paternal obesity at the time of conception can epigenetically alter the paternal germ-line. The paternal germ-line is responsible for regulating their daughters' weight at birth and the potential for their daughter to develop breast cancer.

Furthermore, it was found that modifications to the miRNA expression profile of the male germline is coupled with elevated body weight Additionally, paternal obesity resulted in an increase in the percentage of female offspring developing carcinogen-induced mammary tumors, which is caused by changes to mammary miRNA expression.

Aside from cancer related afflictions associated with the effects of transgenerational epigenetic inheritance, transgenerational epigenetic inheritance has recently been implicated in the progression of pulmonary arterial hypertension (PAH).

Recent studies have found that transgenerational epigenetic inheritance is likely to be involved in the progression of PAH because current therapies for PAH do not repair the irregular phenotypes associated with this disease. Current treatments for PAH have attempted to correct symptoms of PAH with vasodilators and antithrombotic protectors, but neither has effectively alleviated the complications related to the impaired phenotypes associated with PAH.[55] The inability of vasodilators and antithrombotic protectants to correct PAH suggests that the progression of PAH is dependent upon multiple variables, which is likely to be consequent of transgenerational epigenetic inheritance.

Specifically, it is thought that transgenerational epigenetics is linked to the phenotypic changes associated with vascular remodeling. For example, hypoxia during gestation may induce transgenerational epigenetic alterations that could prove to be detrimental during the early phases of fetal development and increase the possibility of developing PAH as an adult Taking the potential effects of transgenerational epigenetics during fetal development into consideration is derived from the fetal origins of adult disease (FOAD) hypothesis, which is related to the concept of fetal programming.

Though hypoxic states could induce the transgenerational epigenetic variance associated with PAH, there is strong evidence to support that a variety of maternal risk factors are linked to the eventual progression of PAH. Such maternal risk factors linked to late-onset PAH includes placental dysfunction, hypertension, obesity, and preeclampsia. These maternal risk factors and environmental stressors coupled with transgenerational epigenetic changes can result in prolonged insult to the signaling pathways associated with the vascular development during fetal stages, thus increasing the likelihood of having PAH.

One study has shown childhood abuse, which is defined as "sexual contact, severe physical abuse and/or severe neglect," leads to epigenetic modifications of glucocorticoid receptor expression Glucocorticoid receptor expression plays a vital role in hypothalamic-pituitary-adrenal (HPA) activity. Additionally, animal experiments have shown that epigenetic changes can depend on mother-infant interactions after birth.

Furthermore, a recent study investigating the correlations between maternal stress in pregnancy and methylation in teenagers/their mothers has found that children of women who were abused during pregnancy were more likely to have methylated glucocorticoid-receptor genes. Thus, children with methylated glucocorticoid-receptor genes experience an altered response to stress, ultimately leading to a higher susceptibility of experiencing anxiety.

Additional studies examining the effects of diethylstilbestrol (DES), which is an endocrine disruptor, have found that the grandchildren (third-generation) of women exposed to DES significantly increased the probability of their grandchildren developing attention-deficit/hyperactivity disorder (ADHD).[60] This is because women exposed to endocrine disruptors, such as DES, during gestation may be linked to multigenerational neurodevelopmental deficits.

Furthermore, animal studies indicate that endocrine

disruptors have a profound impact on germline cells and neurodevelopment. The cause of DES's multigenerational impact is postulated to be the result of biological processes associated with epigenetic reprogramming of the germ line, though this has yet to be determined.

# CHAPTER FOUR

# • Epigenetics and Disease

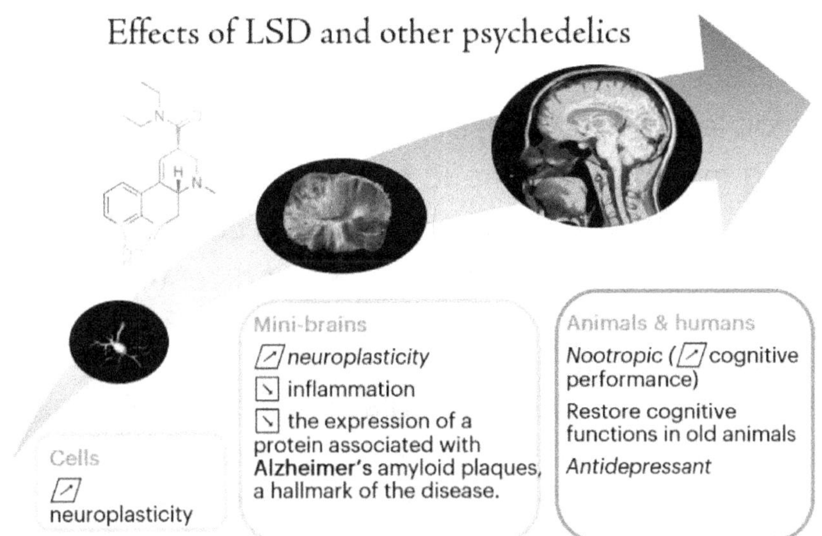



Epigenetics refers to the study of changes in gene function that do not involve changes to the underlying DNA sequence. These changes can affect the way genes are expressed and can lead to the development of various diseases. Epigenetic changes can be caused by environmental factors such as diet, stress, and exposure to toxins, as well as genetic factors.

Epigenetic changes can lead to the development of various diseases, such as cancer, diabetes, and heart disease. For example, epigenetic changes can lead to the silencing of tumor suppressor genes, which can increase the risk of cancer. Similarly, changes in the expression of genes involved in glucose metabolism can contribute to the development of diabetes.

The study of epigenetics is important because it helps us to understand how environmental factors can affect gene expression and lead to the development of disease. By identifying specific epigenetic changes that contribute to the development of disease, researchers can develop new therapies that target these changes and restore normal gene function.

In addition, epigenetic also plays a role in the heritability of certain diseases and traits. Epigenetic marks can be passed down through generations and can affect the risk of disease in future generations. This helps to explain how environmental factors experienced by one generation can affect the health of future generations.

Overall, the field of epigenetics is rapidly advancing, and it holds great promise for improving our understanding of the underlying mechanisms of disease and developing new therapies to prevent and treat various diseases.

## • Cancer

One of the causes of cancer is abnormal genes. Cancer causing genes are called oncogenes and genes that prevent cancer are called tumor suppressor genes. Cancers can occur when the normal genes are not functioning normally. Genes, as you know, are the blueprints to the body. They tell a cell what it will be and what it will do. We could not function if the process did not run well. There is a system in place that is designed to keep good genes running and suppress bad genes. This process is called epigenetics.

Epigenetic changes are modifications to the genome that are heritable during cell division but do not involve a change in DNA sequence. Expression of genes is not regulated by the DNA sequence, which is the same in every cell, but by epigenetic marking and packaging. This process regulates chromatin structure through DNA methylation, histone variants, post-translational modifications, nucleosome positioning factors or chromatin loop and domain organization.

How can this cause cancer? Well, if a tumor suppressor gene is abnormally turned off, or an oncogene is turned on, then cancer (carcinogenesis) can occur. One key is a chemical change to the DNA called methylation. First, we need to define the process to make it clearer.

DNA contains four bases: adenine, guanine, cytosine, thymidine, but there is a fifth base methylated cytosine. DNA methyl-transferase (DNMT) produces methyl-cytosine where cytosines precede guanine (CpG). The CpG areas are not symmetric but clustered in CpG islands located at promoter regions. The promoter region is the region at the beginning of a gene and it controls the start of gene transcription. If the promoter is off, then the gene never is expressed.

Abnormal methylation in cancer has been known for 20 years. Hypo-methylated areas turn on normally silent areas such as virally inserted genes or inactive X-linked genes. Hyper-methylated areas silence tumor suppresser genes.

We know that cancers have abnormal levels of methylation and we know foods can help prevent cancers. Is there a link between foods and epigenetics? Yes!

The study of food nutrients and their effect on disease through epigenetics is known as nutrigenomics. This is a growing field, in fact, it is exploding. A Google search for the term nutrigenomics produces 127,000 entries.

Epidemiologic studies suggest there are bad foods and good foods. BAD: red meat, processed meat, grilled meat, dairy, animal fat, partially hydrogenated fats. Good: Fish, fruits, vegetables, tree nuts, omega-3 fatty acids, whole grains.

You can study the epigenetic effects of bad or good foods.

I'm going to talk about some of the cancer preventing foods and how their mechanisms include epigenetic effects.

Foods with epigenetic effects include green tea, cruciferous vegetables, and grapes. Usually we hear about antioxidants and foods. Antioxidants are important but there are beneficial substances in foods called polyphenols which can affect genes. Of the polyphenols, different forms exist but flavonoids are the most highly cited for health benefits and are found in a variety of vegetables and fruits. Types of flavonoids include flavanols in tea, isothiocyanate in cruciferous vegetables, anthocyanidins in grapes and berries, flavonone in citrus fruits, flavonols in onions, isoflavones (genistein) in soy.

All tea contains polyphenols, but the highest levels are in green and white tea. Green tea has been well studied and appears to have anti-cancer benefits. In China, green tea drinkers are 50% less likely to develop gastric or esophageal cancer (Carcin 2002; 23 (9): 1497), and 2 cups daily added to topical tea extract reversed oral leukoplakia (J. Nutri Biochem 2001; 12 (7): 404).

Green tea has powerful antioxidant effects but it also helps to balance normal methylation in DNA. In fact, one study in esophageal cancer cells demonstrated that EGCG from green tea is able to turn on tumor suppressor genes that had been chemically silenced by methylation (Cancer Research 2003;63:7563).

Cruciferous vegetables include broccoli, cauliflower, kale, Bok choi and their anti-cancer effects have been demonstrated in epidemiologic studies. These powerful vegetables not only induce enzymes that break down carcinogens but they also inhibit DNA methylation allowing tumor suppressor genes to thrive. Inhibiting abnormal methylation also helps cruciferous vegetables to inhibit the cancer causing action of tobacco smoke by preventing the formation of nitrosamine-DNA adducts.

Grapes, which contain reserveratrol, are excellent for heart health and they have anti-cancer activity. Grapes work by preventing the formation or initiation and promotion of cancers. They don't have methylating actions as discussed above but they work by modulation histones.

Histones are the chief protein component of the DNA chain (chromatin). They act as spools for the DNA to wind around which then shortens the length of the DNA to 30,000 times shorter than an unwrapped strand. This process not only allows the long DNA chain to fit into a cell but also plays a role in gene expression because how the genes are wound affects which are exposed and available for turning on or off. Rolling the spool a different way would expose other genes and change their expression.

Histones are modified after translation by acetylation, methylation, phosphorylation, ubiquitination. The changes occur at lysine residues (except for phosphorylation of serine or threonine). When the histone is acetylated the charge is changed and the histone loosens its grip on the DNA strand and the DNA unwinds, exposing the genes to be transcribed, or repaired.

When histone tails (H3,H4) are acetylated, genes are transcribed, when they are deacetylated, genes are turned off. Histone deacetylases work to maintain deacetylated sites.

Resveratrol, found in grapes, activates Sirtuins; SirT1 (Sir2 proteins). There are at least 7 Sir2-like proteins and they are histone deacetylators. Sirtuins are induced in animals during starvation states. They seem to have a life preservation effect. Interestingly, when an animal is starved, it can live longer. When the calorie intake of rodents was decreased by 40% in rodents, they actually lived 50% longer and appear to have fewer chronic diseases. The same benefit occurs when rodents when they are given resveratrol in their diet.

Resveratrol deacetylates histones causing tighter

packing of the chromatin and a lower level of transcription of DNA. This silencing of the DNA is thought to be the mechanism of life prolongation, heart health, and its beneficial actions to prevent cancers. This is why grapes or red wine is beneficial to your health. How much red wine should you drink? No one knows for sure, but any beneficial effects might be negated after two glasses a day because of the alcohol. I wouldn't advise drinking more than this until more is known. The data is very promising, but more research is needed.

Our knowledge of disease expanded in the genomic era due to the human genome project but the study of genes is not enough. Epigenetics is a very important and complicated concept that helps explain how genes are turned on or off. As more studies are completed we will be able to unlock the mechanisms to diseases and produce new therapies that could turn off bad genes and turn on good genes. More importantly, these studies will demonstrate how foods affect your genes and can prevent or reverse diseases or cancers. Nutrigenomics, the study of how food chemicals (nutrients) affect genes, is a growing field and promises to change the way we look at and eat our meals. Some of the most beneficial foods include green tea, cruciferous vegetables and grapes, but don't stop there. The more fruits and vegetables the better when it comes to your health.

## • Neurodegenerative disorders

Neurodegenerative disorders form a group of diseases in which there is a progressive loss of structure or function of neurons or nerve cells in the brain and spinal cord, resulting in progressive degeneration and death of the nerve cells causing problems with movement (ataxia) or with mental functioning (dementia). These disorders are characterized by a standard pathological process involving inflammation; oxidative stress; abnormal depletion or insufficient synthesis of neurotransmitters; and genetic mutations, causing damage to protein synthesis and premature cell death. This results in aggregation or deposit of abnormal protein clumps in various parts of the brain and spinal cord, and characteristic symptoms which help in identifying specific diseases. More than 200 such diseases are listed in this group; the commonly known diseases include Alzheimer's disease (AD), Parkinson's disease (PD), Huntington's disease (HD), Amyotrophic Lateral Sclerosis (ALS), and Ataxias [including Spino-Cerebellar Ataxia (SCA)].

# Neurodegenerative Diseases

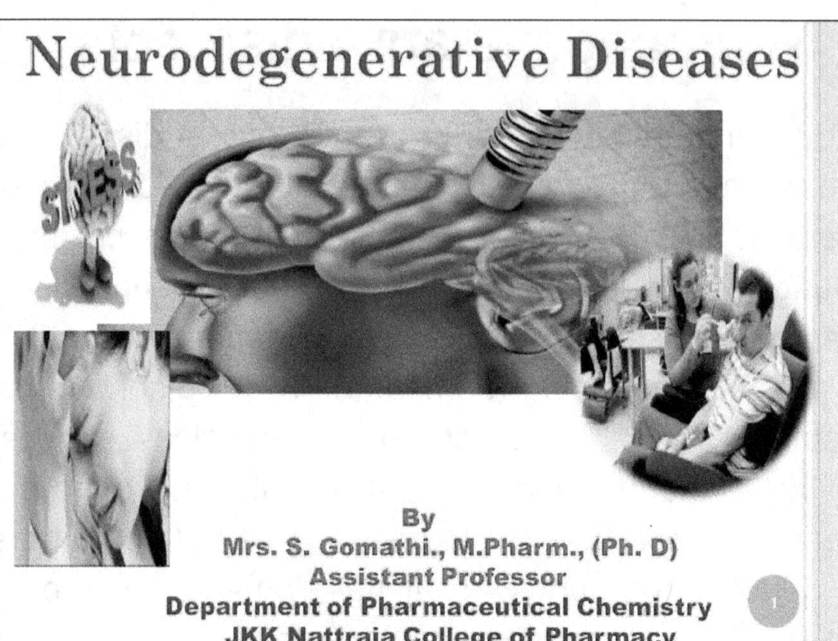

By
Mrs. S. Gomathi., M.Pharm., (Ph. D)
Assistant Professor
Department of Pharmaceutical Chemistry
JKK Nattraja College of Pharmacy
Kumarapalayam  638183

Neurodegenerative disorders are conditions in which cells in the brain break down, causing problems with how people move, think, feel or behave. They are a diverse group of conditions including motor neurone disease, Alzheimer's disease, Parkinson's disease and Huntington's disease.

Our research aims to understand the causes of neurodegenerative disorders and work towards new treatments for these conditions.

**Our research**

Neurodegenerative disorders are associated with cell death in the brain. Cell death could be a direct cause of neurodegenerative disorders or a consequence of other processes that damage brain cells.

## Our researchers are:

Finding genes responsible for neurodegenerative disorders.

Studying how cell death occurs and how it impacts on neurodegenerative disorders.

Developing drugs to block cell death in neurodegenerative disorders.

Investigating how the immune system contributes to

neurodegenerative disorders.

We are also performing research relevant to other conditions with altered brain function, such as:

Studying normal brain development and how this is altered in intellectual disability syndromes.

Exploring how a common parasite changes brain cells and how this could contribute to schizophrenia and bipolar disorder.

## What are neurodegenerative disorders?

Neurodegenerative disorders are conditions that predominantly affect cells in the brain, called neurons.

Neurons are specialised cells that allow the brain to communicate with the rest of the body.When neurons become damaged or die, there is a loss of brain activity leading to problems with movement or mental functioning.

## What are the symptoms of neurodegenerative disorders?

The symptoms of neurodegenerative disorders vary depending on which brain regions are affected.

Some neurodegenerative disorders mainly cause problems with movement (ataxias), while others mainly cause problems with mental functioning (dementias).

Some of the most common neurodegenerative disorders are:

Alzheimer's disease – a form of dementia in which mental functioning, particularly memory, is impaired.

Parkinson's disease – a condition resulting from the degeneration of certain neurons, leading to impaired control of body movements.

Motor neurone disease – a group of diseases in which the neurons that control the muscles degenerate and die, leading to loss of muscle control and eventually paralysis.

Huntington's disease – an inherited neurodegenerative disorder that causes problems with both movement and mental functioning.

Most neurodegenerative disorders develop later in life and are progressive, meaning they lead to increasing disability over time.

## What causes neurodegenerative disorders?

Some neurodegenerative disorders are caused by inherited genetic changes. These disorders run in families: the faulty gene is transmitted from parents to their children. Examples of genetic neurodegenerative disorders include Huntington's disease, and rare cases of motor neurone disease and Alzheimer's disease.

The majority of neurodegenerative disorders are due to a combination of genetic and environmental factors. This makes it difficult to predict who will develop disease.

Specific genetic changes that increase the chance of disease have been identified for some conditions, but in most cases the genetic influences on neurodegenerative disorders are not well understood.

Environmental factors also contribute to neurodegenerative disorders. For example, there is evidence linking Parkinson's disease with long-term exposure to pesticides, toxins and chemicals.

The greatest known risk factor for many neurodegenerative disorders is age. In Australia there are more than 400,000 people living with dementia and around 80,000 people with Parkinson's disease. These figures are likely to rise as the population ages, making neurodegenerative disorders a growing healthcare concern.

## How are neurodegenerative disorders treated?

There are currently no drugs to prevent or cure

neurodegenerative disorders.

Medications to control symptoms can be very effective. Other approaches to manage symptoms and maintain daily activities include physiotherapy, speech pathology, occupational therapy and psychiatry. A multidisciplinary approach is typically applied to improve the quality of life for people with neurodegenerative disorders.

We are committed to research to find much-needed new treatments for neurodegenerative disorders

These conditions are typically brought on by age but not always. Some research shows that these diseases have become more prevalent in recent times, partly due to an increase in the elderly population across the globe.

Neurodegenerative diseases include conditions such as Alzheimer's disease and Parkinson's disease. Neurodegenerative disorders are progressive, which means that they get worse over time. Unfortunately, there's currently no cure, and this progression can't be stopped.

## Symptoms of Neurodegenerative Diseases

Neurodegenerative diseases share a lot of common symptoms. Symptoms of these diseases progress in severity the longer you live with the condition. While medication can help manage and sometimes even slow progression, it can't stop it.

**Some of them include:**

Impaired mental functioning

Loss of muscle control

Taking a longer amount of time to learn new skills

Memory loss

Disorientation

Emotional blunting

Social withdrawal

Hallucinations

Delusions

Depression

Experiencing unwanted thoughts and feelings

Put Your Short-Term Memory to the Test

Identifying Neurodegenerative Diseases

When diagnosing you with a neurodegenerative disease, the first thing your doctor is likely to test is your cognitive function.

A decline in cognitive functioning is a common symptom of all neurodegenerative diseases.1 However, each condition under this umbrella also has its own diagnostic criteria.

Your doctor might also order brain imaging tests like an MRI to confirm a diagnosis. There is ongoing research into the early detection of neurodegenerative diseases.

A test is done for the presence of microRNAs (miRNAs), which might contain potential biomarkers for neurodegenerative disease. A miRNA is a single-stranded molecule that plays a role in regulating gene expression.

## Causes of Neurodegenerative Diseases

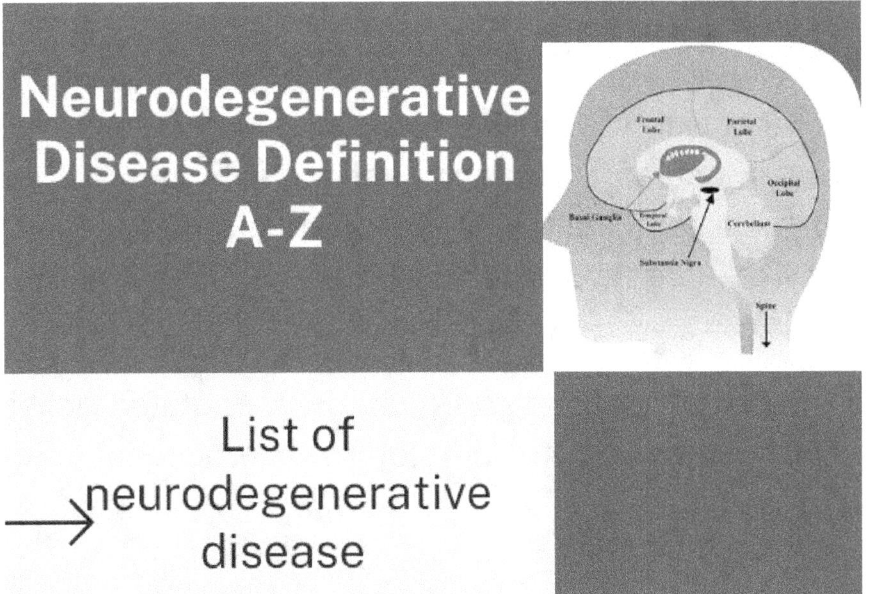

Below are some of the causes of neurodegenerative diseases.

Neuronal Damage

Neurodegenerative diseases are thought to be caused by damage to neurons in your brain. Neurons make up your nervous system which includes your brain and spinal cord.

Unlike some parts of your body, when a neuron gets damaged, it's unable to replace itself. And, as you age, these neurons die. In fact, as you get older, the brain shrinks.

Neurodegenerative diseases cause these neurons to die. When these neurons die, you experience symptoms that affect your mental functioning, movement, and ability to breathe or speak.

## Environmental and Genetic Factors

It's not very clear what brings on most neurodegenerative diseases. Most of these conditions are thought to be caused by a combination of environmental and genetic factors like long-term exposure to toxins and certain chemicals.

In some cases, relatives can pass down mutated genes that can cause you to develop a neurodegenerative disease.

## Abnormal Proteins

Abnormal proteins in the brain have also been linked to many neurodegenerative diseases. These abnormal proteins can cause nerve cells in your brain to die. With Alzheimer's disease, a protein known as beta-amyloid has been linked to the development of the condition.

Synuclein is another abnormal protein that has been observed in the brains of people with Lewy body dementia, Parkinson's disease, and multiple system atrophy.9

## Risk Factors for Developing Neurodegenerative Diseases

Certain risk factors can increase your risk of developing a neurodegenerative disease. The most significant risk factor for developing a neurodegenerative disease is old age.

As you age, nerve cells in your brain are more likely to die. These factors include having conditions such as cardiovascular diseases or experiencing brain trauma. Other factors include:

- Smoking

- Poor diet

- Alcohol use disorder

- Depression

- Brain tumor

- Stroke

- Mental Health Effects of a Stroke

# Types of Neurodegenerative Diseases

There are many different forms of neurodegenerative diseases. Some of the most common are detailed below.

## Alzheimer's Disease

Alzheimer's disease is one of the most common neurodegenerative diseases in the United States today. Research shows that around 6.2 million people may have the condition as of 2022.11

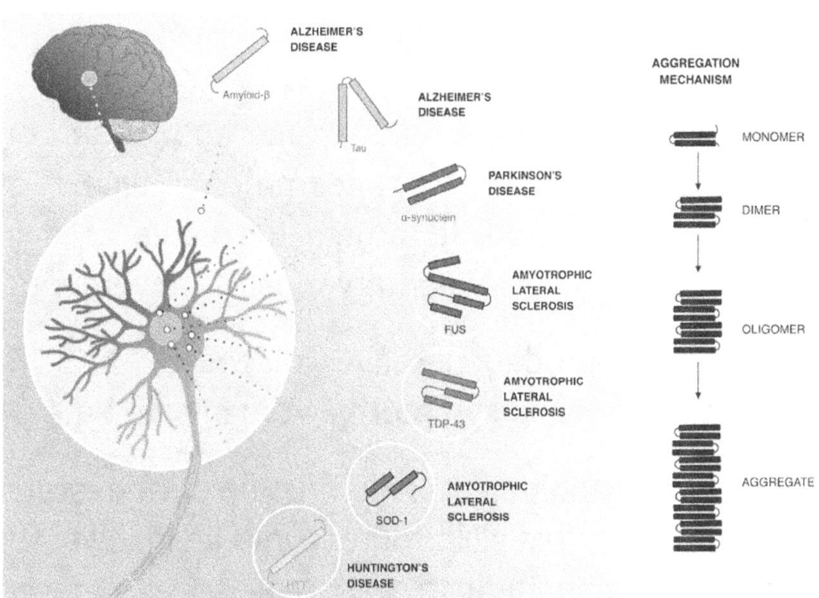

## Common symptoms include:

- Getting lost

- Memory loss

- Personality changes

There are two forms of this disorder: late-onset Alzheimer's disease and early-onset Alzheimer's disease. The former is more common and affects people over the age of 60. The latter is rare and can develop in people who are between the ages of 30 and 60.13

**Amyotrophic Lateral Sclerosis**

Amyotrophic lateral sclerosis (ALS), also known as Lou Gehrig's disease, is an uncommon type of neurodegenerative disease. It targets the nerve cells in your brain that control your voluntary muscle movement.

As with most neurodegenerative diseases, ALS is progressive, which means symptoms worsen over time.

Early signs of the condition include muscle stiffness and weakness. With time, this will progress into an inability for a person with the condition to walk, eat, speak or even breathe.

# Huntington's Disease

Huntington's disease is a condition that causes you to lose control over your body. It also causes cognitive decline.

## Early symptoms of the disorder include:

- Depression

- Slight involuntary movements

- Irritability

- Poor decision-making skills

As the condition progresses, more severe symptoms such as difficulty walking and swallowing, increased involuntary movements and personality changes develop.15

## Lewy Body Dementia

Lewy body dementia is a condition that's caused by abnormal deposits of a protein in your brain. The alpha-synuclein protein causes chemical changes in the brain that lead to cognitive decline and mood and behavior changes.

This condition is often mistaken for Parkinson's disease

because both conditions share several common symptoms. Common symptoms of Lewy body dementia include visual hallucinations and confusion.16

## Parkinson's Disease

Parkinson's disease is a condition that progressively causes difficulty in movement in people living with it. Early signs of the condition include tremors.

As the disease progresses, your muscles become stiffer, and movement becomes more difficult. While the condition is primarily marked by difficulty with movement, it also causes a loss of cognitive function.

## Treatment for Neurodegenerative Diseases

Unfortunately, there's currently no cure for neurodegenerative diseases. They are typically treated with a combination of medication and psychotherapy.

The exact combination and form of drugs depend on the form of neurodegenerative disease one has been diagnosed with.

Treatment for each form of the neurodegenerative disease varies. However, treatment typically focuses on alleviating symptoms of the condition.

## Research Is Ongoing

Over the last few decades, cutting-edge research has made leaps and strides in developing new innovative medications for treating neurodegenerative diseases. For example, there is ongoing research into using immunotherapy to treat Alzheimer's disease symptoms.

Medications help manage the physical and mental symptoms of neurodegenerative diseases. Unfortunately, these diseases are progressive, and there are currently no medications that can help to slow down the progression of their symptoms

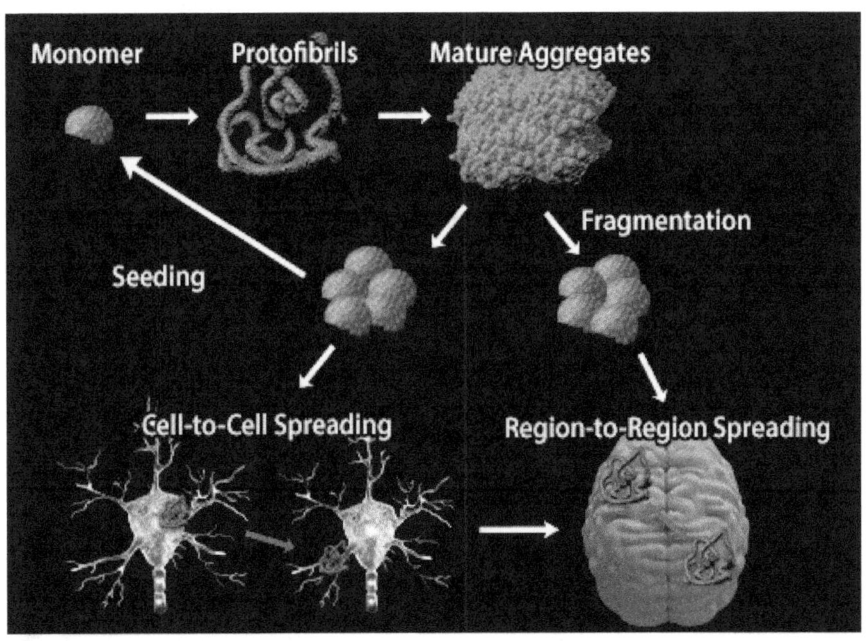

Neurodegenerative disorders are a group of progressive conditions that affect the structure and function of the brain and spinal cord. These disorders include Alzheimer's disease, Parkinson's disease, Huntington's disease, and Amyotrophic lateral sclerosis (ALS). They are characterized by the gradual loss of nerve cells and the deterioration of cognitive and motor function. The causes of these disorders are not well understood, but they may involve a combination of genetic, environmental, and lifestyle factors. There is currently no cure for neurodegenerative disorders, but treatments are available to manage symptoms and slow the progression of the disease.

# • Metabolic and cardiovascular disorders

Metabolism is one of the many critical systems running in our bodies. It is surely working all the time, but boosting it will make perfect effect on your health and may your health goals closer much faster.

## About the Report

This report will not dive into chemistry of metabolism or more specific sub-categories of metabolism. The key of the report is to give short basic presentation of metabolism and introduce some Quick Tricks for boosting your personal metabolism process to give better and faster results for Weight Lose and Better Health. Some of the tricks are even fun to use!

## Metabolism - the Key

"Metabolism is the set of life-sustaining chemical transformations within the cells of living organisms. These enzyme-catalyzed reactions allow organisms to grow and reproduce, maintain their structures, and respond to their environments." (Wikipedia definition)

What does that mean for my health and weight lose? Everything! Metabolism is the process that drives the fat out of your body and also drives all necessary supplements for better health into your body. Metabolism and other organic chemistry of human body are very interesting subjects of their own, but in this report let's just focus on improving our metabolism process.

Having a high level of metabolism enables one to maintain burn fat and lose weight fast with the least amount of activity. Metabolism is the rate by which the body produces and consumes energy and calories to support life.

There are several factors that affect the metabolism of a person, such as the amount of muscle tissue, the frequency of the meals one consumes, genetics, stress levels, personal diet and activity levels.

Metabolism slows down due to loss of muscle because of not enough physical activity, the tendency of the body to cannibalize its own tissue because nutritional value of the food is not enough to sustain it, and the decrease of physical activity that comes naturally with old age.

**Luckily, there are several ways to boost the metabolism of your body:**

• Sleep more

• Increase water intake

- Increase muscle mass

- Eat smart

- Relax

- Stay focused and motivated!

# Sleep more

Start with sleeping more. Enough amount of good sleep changes between people, but last researches have pointed out that one should sleep even some 8 hours per night. Sleeping under 6 hours increases the risk of several disorders for your body and slows down metabolism.

When you are tired, everything is difficult, you make bad decisions. You envy for fast carbohydrates and fat in your food. You eat for your tiredness.

Muscles are regenerated during the rest and especially while sleeping. Also brain needs to rest and sleeping improves also your memory. There are so many benefits of good sleep, so make your sleeping better first.

### Increase water income

The average adult human body is 50-65% of water. Water is basic element of the cells what we are built of.

Our body is losing water all time by skin evaporation,

breathing, urine and feces. These losses must be replaced or we will be suffering about dehydration.

Water also flushes out toxins that are produced whenever the body burns fat. Majority of bodily functions involves water, and lack of water causes the body system's operations to decrease its speed, and produces unneeded stress as a result.

## Increase muscle mass

Let's go exercising!

Build up on lean, mean body mass. It is only natural that metabolism decreases along with age, but it is possible to counter the effects. The amount of muscle a person has is a very strong determinant in the ability to burn calories and shed fat.

So it goes without saying that exercise is essential. Build strength and resistance by working out at least twice a week, preferably with weights. Do easy exercises in between workouts. Simple tasks such as walking the dog and using the stairs in place of the elevator can already take off calories. The key is to match the amount of eating to the amount of activity one has. Here are some guidelines in getting the right exercise:

## For strength training

• Increase the amount of repetitions of a particular exercise.

• Add the level of resistance

• Utilize advance exercise techniques if possible

**For cardiovascular training**

• Insert intervals between exercises

• Perform cross-training and combine the exercises

• Add up on resistance and speed

**Eat smart**

Eat breakfast. A lot of people are ignoring the fact that breakfast is the most important meal of the day. Surprisingly, the ones who eat breakfast are thinner than the ones who do not. Metabolism can slow down considerably if breakfast is taken during mid-morning or if one waits until the afternoon to eat.

Avoid sugar. Sugar enables the body to store fat. It is recommended that a person consumes food that helps sustain an even level of blood-sugar. Additionally, progressive exercise 2-3 times a week should be in order to stabilize blood sugar.

Eat spicy foods. Hot cuisine with peppers can increase

metabolism.

Eat smaller meals. It is advisable to consume 4 to 6 small meals that are timed 2 to 3 hours apart.

Never skip meals. People tend to skip meals in order to lose weight, which is a big mistake since it slows down metabolism.

Plan meals in detail. Always prepare the right amount of food to be consumed at the designated intervals. Do not commit the mistake of eating meals in sporadic patterns.

Do not get stuck with meat and potatoes any more. It is nowadays common knowledge that vegetables, fruits, whole grains, nuts, and fish are the best for you. Remember to have enough protein in your diet.

**Relax**

Ditch the stress! Be it physical or emotional, stress triggers the release of a steroid called cortisol, which decreases metabolism. Also, people tend to eat excessively when stressed.

Don't worry about changing your eating, training, water drinking or any other new habits immediately. Decide to make a change, do little steps after another, be focused on your goals and relax. You will achieve your goals.

## Stay focused and motivated

Achieving the desired body weight or other goal is never impossible if one has the determination and patience needed to stabilize the metabolism level. A person needs to realize that eating right and working out is not just a passing fancy, but a way of life.

## Start now and keep going

This report gave you some fast ideas how to improve metabolism of your body. Take some of the advice, decide to take first step and take it! Do not try to fix everything in one step, take it piece by piece. And enjoy your path for better health.

## Life is for living!

Hopefully you got new ideas from the article!

This article is about tips for boosting metabolism, the ultimate key for weight lose and overall health improvement. The article was written by Mark Twig, who is also known as Best healthmate, your health coach and mentor.

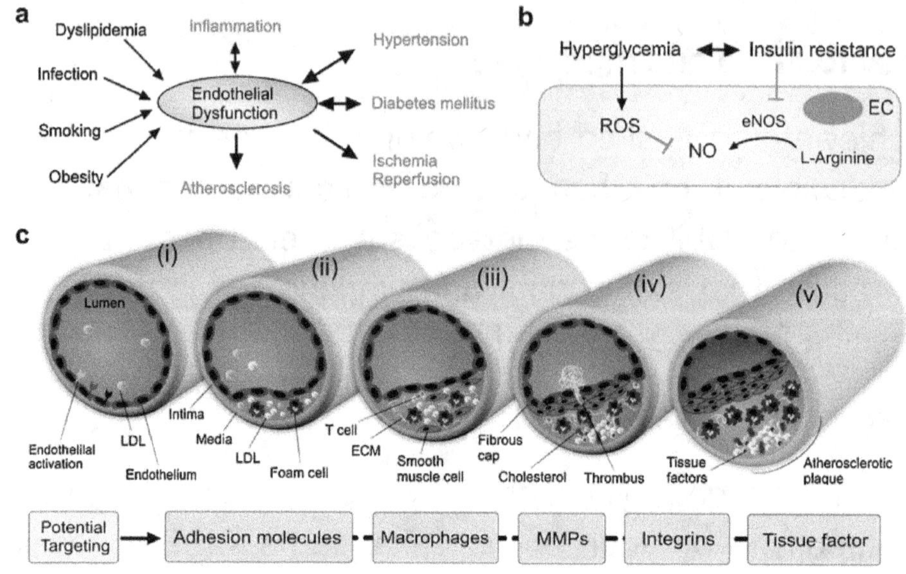



Epigenetics is the study of heritable changes in gene expression that occur without changes to the underlying DNA sequence. These changes can be caused by a variety of factors, including environmental exposures, diet, and lifestyle. Metabolic and cardiovascular disorders, such as obesity, diabetes, and heart disease, have been linked to epigenetic changes in several key genes and pathways.

Obesity is a complex disorder that is influenced by both genetic and environmental factors. Studies have shown that epigenetic changes in genes involved in appetite regulation and energy metabolism can lead to increased body weight and obesity. For example, methylation of the FTO gene, which is involved in appetite regulation, has been associated with increased body weight and obesity. Similarly, methylation of the PPAR-γ gene, which regulates energy metabolism, has been linked to obesity and metabolic disorders.

Diabetes is a metabolic disorder characterized by high blood sugar levels. Epigenetic changes in genes involved in insulin production and glucose metabolism have been linked to the development of diabetes. For example, methylation of the insulin receptor gene has been associated with reduced insulin sensitivity and increased risk of diabetes. Similarly, methylation of the glucokinase gene, which regulates glucose metabolism, has been linked to diabetes and metabolic disorders.

Heart disease is a leading cause of death worldwide. Epigenetic changes in genes involved in inflammation, cholesterol metabolism, and blood pressure regulation have been linked to the development of heart disease. For example, methylation of the LEP gene, which regulates appetite and body weight, has been associated with increased risk of heart disease. Similarly, methylation of the PCSK9 gene, which regulates cholesterol metabolism, has been linked to heart disease and metabolic disorders.

Overall, epigenetics plays a significant role in the development of metabolic and cardiovascular disorders. Understanding the underlying epigenetic mechanisms involved in these disorders can lead to the development of new diagnostic and therapeutic strategies for these diseases.

# • Mental illness

Mental illness, such as depression, schizophrenia, and bipolar disorder, also have a strong epigenetic component. Studies have shown that epigenetic changes in genes involved in brain development, neurotransmitter regulation, and stress response can contribute to the development of mental illness.

Depression is a complex mental disorder characterized by feelings of sadness, loss of interest, and a lack of energy. Epigenetic changes in genes involved in neurotransmitter regulation, such as the serotonin transporter gene, have been linked to depression. Studies have shown that methylation of the serotonin transporter gene can lead to reduced expression of the gene and increased risk of depression.

Schizophrenia is a chronic mental disorder characterized by hallucinations, delusions, and disordered thinking. Epigenetic changes in genes involved in brain development and neurotransmitter regulation have been linked to schizophrenia. For example, methylation of the

DISC1 gene, which is involved in brain development, has been associated with increased risk of schizophrenia. Similarly, methylation of the dopamine receptor gene has been linked to schizophrenia and other mental disorders.

Bipolar disorder is a mental disorder characterized by episodes of mania and depression. Epigenetic changes in genes involved in stress response and neurotransmitter regulation have been linked to bipolar disorder. For example, methylation of the FKBP5 gene, which regulates the stress response, has been associated with increased risk of bipolar disorder. Similarly, methylation of the serotonin receptor gene has been linked to bipolar disorder and other mental disorders.

Overall, mental illness is a complex and multifactorial disease that is influenced by a combination of genetic, environmental, and epigenetic factors. Understanding the epigenetic mechanisms involved in mental illness can lead to the development of new diagnostic and therapeutic strategies for these disorders.

# CHAPTER FIVE

# • Epigenetic and the Environment

Epigenetics is the study of heritable changes in gene expression that occur without changes to the underlying DNA sequence. These changes can be caused by a variety of factors, including environmental exposures. The environment plays a crucial role in shaping an individual's epigenetic profile, and can have long-lasting effects on health and disease.

Environmental exposures such as diet, toxins, and stress can cause epigenetic changes that can lead to chronic diseases such as cancer, heart disease, and mental illness. For example, a diet high in processed foods and sugar can cause epigenetic changes in genes involved in metabolism and inflammation, leading to an increased risk of obesity and heart disease. Similarly, exposure to toxins such as pesticides and heavy metals can cause epigenetic changes in genes involved in cancer development, leading to an increased risk of cancer.

Stress is also a significant environmental factor that can cause epigenetic changes. Chronic stress can lead to epigenetic changes in genes involved in the stress response, leading to an increased risk of mental illness and chronic diseases. For example, methylation of the FKBP5 gene, which regulates the stress response, has been associated with increased risk of depression and anxiety.

Epigenetic changes caused by environmental exposures can also be passed down from one generation to the next. This is known as transgenerational epigenetics. For example, studies have shown that exposure to toxins such as pesticides can cause epigenetic changes in sperm and eggs, leading to an increased risk of chronic diseases in the next generation.

Overall, the environment plays a crucial role in shaping an individual's epigenetic profile, and can have long-lasting effects on health and disease. Understanding the epigenetic mechanisms involved in environmental exposures can lead to the development of new strategies for preventing and treating chronic diseases.

# THE EFFECTS OF ENVIRONMENTAL FACTORS ON THE EPIGENOME

To understand the impact of the environment on the

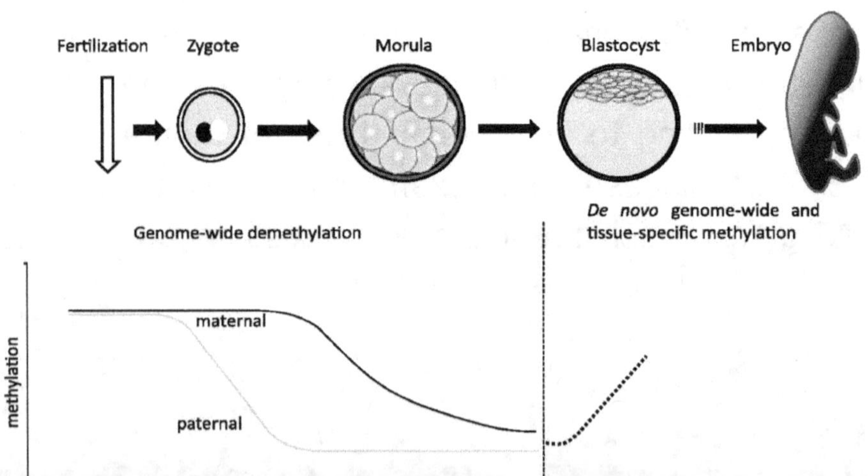

epigenotype, it is necessary to consider two scenarios: embryonic development and adult life. The need to differentiate between prenatal and postnatal life arises from the differential impact that an epigenetic change can have on the organism. In principle, the epigenetic changes occurring during embryonic development will have a much greater impact on the overall epigenetic status of the organism because, as they can be transmitted over consecutive mitotic divisions, alterations occurring in single embryonic stem cells will affect many more cells than those occurring in adult stem and/or somatic cells during postnatal development. Although this possibility is plausible, it remains to be firmly established. In the final analysis, the type of change and the genomic location of the change(s) may dictate the clinical significance of the epigenetic changes, along with genetic background and random other variables.

## The Impact of the Environment on the Epigenome During Embryonic Development

The environmental conditions in the uterus can determine phenotypic alterations in the offspring that, since they persist throughout life, can give rise to stable changes in gene expression. Recent studies suggest that such stable gene regulation can be mediated, at least in part, by epigenetic mechanisms. In principle, the environmental conditions during embryonic development must be primarily determined by two factors: 1) the specific phenotypes of the mother and the placenta, which determine characteristics, such as the size of the uterus and the availability of nutrients; and 2) the mother's lifestyle, which determines the environmental factors to which the embryo is exposed (Fig. 3, Table 1). Although little is currently known about how the phenotypes of the mother and the placenta can affect the epigenotypes of the offspring [it has been suggested that maternal obesity can lead to specific epigenetic alterations of the offspring (109)], there is a great deal of information about how the environmental conditions of the mother can affect specific epigenetic factors of their offspring.

The best studied environmental condition of the mother affecting the epigenotype of the offspring is maternal diet. A good example of how this can affect specific epigenetic pathways of the offspring comes from agouti mice. The agouti alleles regulate the production of pigment in individual hair follicles. Yellow and mottled mice are obese and prone to diabetes and cancer, in contrast to fully agouti mice, known as pseudoagoutis, which are lean and nondiabetic. The phenotype of the agouti mice depends on the expression of the agouti protein, which is regulated by the DNA methylation status of a repeated DNA region at the agouti promoter (66), and, interestingly, methyl donor supplementation of female mice before and during pregnancy permanently increases tissue-specific DNA methylation of the agouti gene in offspring (106–108). In keeping with this observation, in utero exposure to a high-fat diet modifies the methylation pattern of leptin and ER promoters in rats (64, 114). Interestingly, maternal diet-dependent methylation changes at the ER promoter boost expression of this gene with aging and, consequently, prompt a higher incidence of tumors in offspring (114). A high-fat diet during pregnancy has also been linked to genomewide and locus-specific methylation changes in the placenta (C. Junien, personal communication).

Other examples of epigenetic modulation in response to environmental factors include the epigenetic downregulation of genes involved in pancreatic B-cell function in abnormal intrauterine environments (89) and the specific DNA methylation profiles of offspring associated with maternal diet (60, 61). Lillycrop and colleagues have shown that, either feeding a protein-restricted diet to pregnant rats and mice, or exposing them to undernutrition, causes stable changes to the epigenetic regulation of glucocorticoid receptor and peroxisomal proliferator-activated receptor-α genes in the livers of juvenile (60, 61) and adult (17) offspring. Interestingly, diet-dependent epigenetic changes are associated with altered messenger RNA expression of these genes and their target genes.

The role of maternal diet in establishing epigenetic marks has recently been confirmed at the genomewide level by Sinclair and colleagues (90). Using restriction landmark genomic scanning, they analyzed the methylation status of 1,400 CpG sites in the offspring of mature female sheep in response to the restriction of the supply of specific B vitamins and methionine from the periconceptional diet (74). They found that the offspring from vitamin-restricted maternal diets had numerous phenotypic alterations, such as increased body mass, altered immune responses to antigenic challenge, insulin resistance, and elevated blood pressure. In addition, 4% of the CpG sites analyzed featured altered methylation, which suggests that specific maternal diets can lead to widespread epigenetic alterations to DNA methylation in offspring and modify adult health-related phenotypes (90).

In humans, it has also recently been found that maternal diet may have an important role in establishing the long-term epigenotype of offspring (94). Tobi and colleagues (94) showed that individuals who were prenatally exposed to famine during the Dutch Hunger Winter exhibited less DNA methylation of the imprinted IGF2 gene 6 decades later compared with their unexposed, same-sex siblings.

The epigenetic alterations were established during periconceptional exposure, thereby supporting the concept that very early mammalian development is a crucial period for establishing and maintaining epigenetic marks. This work provides evidence that environmental conditions early on in human life can cause epigenetic changes that persist throughout life. Future studies will decipher the functional role of these epigenetic marks acquired during embryonic development in the establishment of specific phenotypes during adult life.

## The Relationship Between Environment and Epigenetics During Adult Life

The effect of specific environmental factors on the epigenetic status of adult organisms has been widely reported (Table 1) (30, 32). However, the precise molecular mechanisms by which the environment can alter the epigenetic marks are still poorly understood and represent a fascinating field of study.

To understand how environmental factors can affect the epigenotype of an organism, it is important to take into account that higher organisms are composed of multiple tissues and that, as epigenetic status is tissue or cell specific, the effects of environmental factors on the epigenotype of an organism can depend on the tissue type (i.e., because the specific epigenetic status of a tissue makes this tissue more resistant to environmentally induced epigenetic alteration). The degree of exposure of a tissue to a specific environmental factor can also determine its ability to induce specific epigenetic alterations within that tissue. For instance, it is easy to imagine that, if UV radiation has a specific effect on a particular epigenetic factor, then this would be much more evident in skin, since this is exposed to solar radiation, than in muscle, which is not.

In humans, the environmental factors that may affect epigenetic status during adult life can be divided into four groups: diet, living place and/or workplace, pharmacological treatments, and unhealthy habits (Fig. 3).

One of the most obvious examples of how the type of diet can affect epigenetic factors is folate intake. Folic acid (vitamin B9) is important for epigenetics, because it is necessary for the remethylation of homocysteine, a key chemical reaction in the metabolic pathway that systematizes S-adenosyl methionine, the methyl donor group of the histone and DNA methylation reactions. The amount of dietary folate intake may be associated with the epigenetic status of the organism (51, 55), and, interestingly, deficiencies in dietary folate result in numerous health alterations that are most evident when they occur during embryonic development (75). Methionine, another dietary compound involved in the metabolic pathway that synthesizes S-adenosyl methionine, is also thought to be involved in epigenetic-dependent hepatic diseases (5). Selenium is a dietary substance that modifies the epigenetic status of an organism at the DNA methylation and histone modification levels (113). Moreover, it has been proposed that cancer prevention by selenium may be mediated by its epigenetic effects (113). Certain dietary polyphenols, such as (-)-epigallocatechin 3-gallate from green tea and genistein from soybean are also thought to prevent cancer by means of epigenetic mechanisms (28). Recently, other substances occurring naturally in some foods, like butyrate in cheeses, diallyl disulphide in garlic, and sulphoraphane in broccoli, have been identified as HDAC inhibitors, and a putative role for some of these has been proposed in cancer chemoprevention through the disruption of the uncontrolled progression of cell cycle or by the induction of apoptosis via increased acetylation and derepression of genes, such as P21 and BAX (18, 23). The effect of diet on the epigenetic status of an organism can be so important that it has even been described that a high-fat diet can be associated with promoter DNA hypermethylation of specific tumor-suppressor genes (15).

Although it seems obvious that, if epigenetic factors can be altered by dietary compounds, then they should also be susceptible to alteration by pharmacological substances; the evidence for the latter is limited. One example is diethylstilbestrol, a drug used by millions of pregnant women to prevent miscarriages and many other disorders in pregnancy, which is currently know to be associated with an increased risk of breast cancer, clear cell adenocarcinoma of the vagina and cervix, and reproductive anomalies (100). Interestingly, it has been proposed that the dramatic health effects of diethylstilbestrol can be mediated by epigenetic mechanisms, since this drug has been shown to alter expression of DNA methyltransferases and methylation of genomic DNA (34, 83). Another example is sodium valproate, an anticonvulsant classically used to treat some mental disorders that is now a well-known and potent inhibitor of HDACs (101). Procaine, a drug that was used in the past as a local anesthetic, is now known to induce DNA demethylation (102). Another example is the antituberculosis drug pyrazinamide, which has recently been shown to induce a decrease in cytosine DNA methylation of long-interspersed nucleotide element-1 and aberrant promoter hypermethylation of p16(INK4A) in rats (57). Several antibiotics have also been shown to induce significant epigenetic alterations. For instance, the anthracycline antibiotic doxorubicin is known to induce conditional apoptosis in cancer cells by the inhibition of the DNA methyltransferase DNMT1 (115).

The living place and/or workplace can determine the level of exposure to many environmental factors that are potentially able to alter epigenetic status. For example, it is obvious that the chemical and xenobiotic composition of the atmosphere and water in a city is different from that in a rural environment. Although it is not entirely certain that these environmental factors are responsible for epigenetic alterations, strong associations among them have been found. One of the best examples of these is the recent observation that, in pleural tissues, at least 24 CpG loci have asbestos-related alterations in methylation, all of which featured increases in methylation (21). Other types of chemical entities that are known to alter DNA methylation levels are metal ions. For instance, the environmental pollutants chromium (87), cadmium (93), and nickel (80) have been shown to reduce methylation levels by inhibiting the activity of DNA methyltransferases. In the case of nickel, carcinogenic nickel compounds can reduce global histone H4 acetylation and increase histone H3 lysine 9 dimethylation at the promoter level, repressing expression of specific genes (20). Other chemicals and xenobiotics to which organisms may be exposed can also change

DNA methylation at a global and/or local level. These include bisphenol A (62), used in the plastics industry, and vinclozolin (4), a fungicide used in vineyards. These molecules are considered to be endocrine disruptors and have been convincingly related to DNA methylation alteration of specific promoters, developmental disorders, and tumorigenesis.

Unhealthy habits, such as alcohol and tobacco consumption and drug abuse, can also alter specific epigenetic factors. Indeed, one of the best current examples of how environmental factors can alter the epigenetic status of an organism is the promoter hypermethylation of tumor-suppressor genes that occurs in nontumorigenic lung tissues of smokers, but not in the corresponding tissues of nonsmokers (8). The relationship between tobacco use and alterations of DNA methylation was recently confirmed by Christensen and colleagues (21), who reported that, in lung tissues, smoking status (smoker vs. never smoker) is associated with altered methylation at 138 CpG loci. Interestingly, these authors also showed that, in adult blood cells, increasing pack-years of smoking was significantly associated with MLH1 and RIPK3 methylation, which suggests that tissues less exposed to cigarette smoke are also prone to smoking-dependent epigenetic alterations. The effect of alcohol consumption on epigenetic factors in humans has been much less extensively studied. One of the few published studies describes how the HERP gene is significantly downregulated by promoter DNA hypermethylation in patients with alcohol dependence compared with healthy controls (13) and that over 30 CpG loci have significantly altered methylation in never-drinkers compared with drinkers (21). However, it has been widely reported that chronic alcohol feeding in rats results in many epigenetic alterations. For instance, chronic ethanol feeding causes the inhibition of the ubiquitin proteasome pathway in the nucleus, which leads to changes in the turnover of transcriptional factors, histone-modifying enzymes, and, therefore, altered epigenetic mechanisms (6, 71).

The abuse of some drugs has also been shown to alter specific epigenetic factors. Indeed, cannabinoids, heroin, and cocaine have been shown to produce deep epigenetic alterations (33).

The best studied epigenetic alterations caused by drug abuse are those caused by cocaine. Maternal cocaine administration in mice is known to alter DNA methylation and gene expression in hippocampus neurons of neonatal and prepubertal offspring (69). In addition, gene regulation by the HMT G9a has an essential role in cocaine-induced plasticity (63), and HDAC inhibitors decrease cocaine self-administration in rats (79). These observations suggest that a number of the physiological effects of cocaine in vivo are mediated by epigenetic mechanisms. Further research is needed to determine the real impact of the abuse of other drugs, such as cannabinoids and heroin, on the epigenome of the organism.

Although it is evident that most of the substances described above can alter specific epigenetic factors, it should be stressed that it is not known whether all of them can be considered authentic epigenetic modifiers, because it has not yet been demonstrated whether the epigenetic modifications that they induce are stable over time.

# • Environmental influences on epigenetic

Environmental influences on epigenetic can be broadly classified into two categories, namely exogenous and endogenous.

Exogenous environmental impacts are defined as outside elements that can alter epigenetic patterns, such as nutrition, poisons, and pollutants. Inflammation and metabolism-related genes, for instance, might undergo epigenetic modifications as a result of a diet high in processed foods and sugar, which increases the risk of obesity and heart disease. Similar epigenetic modifications in cancer-related genes can be brought on by exposure to chemicals like pesticides and heavy metals, increasing the risk of developing cancer.

Endogenous environmental impacts are internal elements that can alter epigenetic patterns, such as stress, infection, and inflammation. For instance, persistent stress can alter the epigenetic state of genes that are involved in the stress response, increasing the risk of mental illness and chronic illnesses.

Similar to how inflammation and infection can alter the epigenetic state of immune response genes, increasing the likelihood of developing chronic illnesses.

It's also crucial to remember that genetic and environmental impacts on epigenetics can work together to influence the epigenetic profile of an individual. For instance, research has demonstrated that environmental influences like nutrition and exercise can alter a person's genetic propensity toward obesity. Similar to how environmental factors like being exposed to poisons and pollutants can change a person's genetic propensity for cancer.

Epigenetic influences from the environment are generally complex and multifaceted, and they can have a long-lasting impact on health and disease. The discovery of novel approaches for the prevention and treatment of chronic diseases can result from a better understanding of the epigenetic pathways connected to environmental exposures.

# • Epigenetic and aging

Epigenetics is the study of changes in gene activity that do not involve changes to the underlying DNA sequence. These changes can be caused by a variety of factors, including environmental exposures, diet, and aging.

Aging is a complex and multifactorial process that is influenced by both genetic and environmental factors. Epigenetic changes play a significant role in aging by altering gene expression, which can lead to changes in cellular function and the development of age-related diseases.

One example of an epigenetic change that occurs with aging is the accumulation of DNA methylation, which is a process by which methyl groups are added to the DNA molecule. This can lead to the suppression of gene expression and changes in cellular function.

Another example is Histone modification, which are changes in the structure of histone proteins that help to control gene expression. As we age, these modifications can lead to the repression of certain genes and the activation of others, leading to changes in cellular function and the development of age-related diseases.

Overall, epigenetics plays a critical role in aging by influencing the expression of genes and the development of age-related diseases. Understanding the mechanisms of epigenetic changes in aging may help to develop new strategies for preventing or treating age-related diseases.

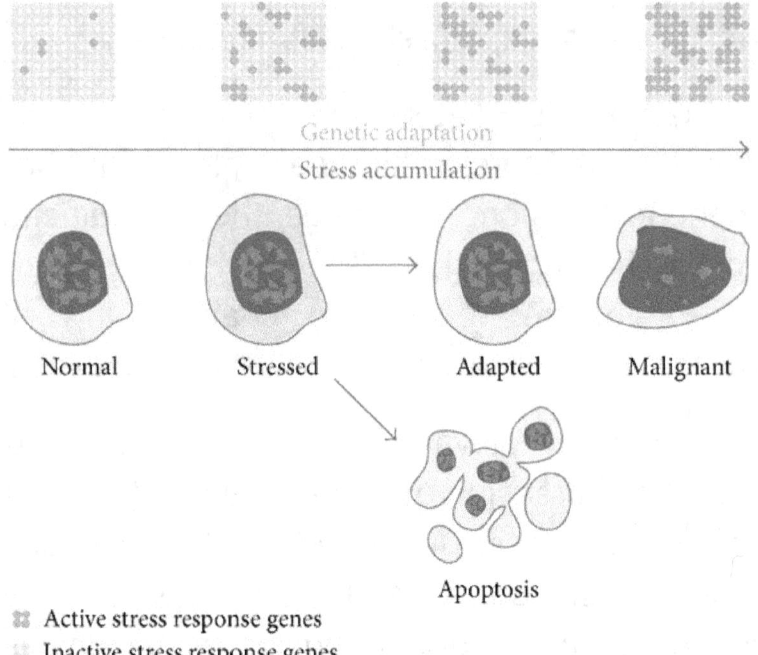



# • Epigenetic responses to stress

Stress is a well-known environmental factor that can lead to epigenetic changes in the body. Stress can activate signaling pathways that lead to changes in the expression of genes, which in turn can affect cellular function and lead to the development of various diseases.

One example of an epigenetic change that occurs in response to stress is the alteration of DNA methylation patterns. Stress can lead to increased DNA methylation in certain genes, which can suppress their expression and lead to changes in cellular function.

Another example is Histone modification, which occurs in response to stress. Stress can lead to changes in the structure of histone proteins, which can affect the accessibility of DNA and alter gene expression.

Stress can also affect the expression of microRNAs (miRNA), which are small non-coding RNAs that regulate gene expression. Stress can lead to changes in the expression of miRNAs, which can in turn lead to changes in the expression of target genes and affect cellular function.

stress can lead to a wide range of epigenetic changes that affect gene expression and cellular function. These changes can contribute to the development of various diseases, including mental disorders and cardiovascular diseases. Understanding the mechanisms of epigenetic changes in response to stress may help to develop new strategies for preventing or treating stress-related diseases.

# Level 1: epigenetic components of stress signaling

Investment into stress defense, alongside constitutive morphological and metabolic survival equipment and seasonal adaptations, expends plants' general resources and therefore should be restricted to the actual occurrence of stressful situations. Plants use a range of different sensing and signaling mechanisms to induce dynamic stress responses only when challenged. Signaling includes mainly the hormones salicylic acid (SA), jasmonic acid (JA) and ethylene upon biotic stress, and abscisic acid (ABA) in case of abiotic stress (reviewed in [1]). Nevertheless, there is growing evidence that noncoding and siRNAs and the proteins generating or binding them are involved in stress-signaling and can subsequently induce transcriptional or posttranscriptional gene silencing (TGS or PTGS, respectively). These principles are described in the review by Wierzbicki (this issue).

There are many examples of differential siRNA, miRNA or ncRNA expression upon stress [2]. The recent identification of a mutated NRPD2 gene responsible for constitutive overexpression of a SA-inducible gene provided a mechanistic link between stress signaling and elements of the RNA directed DNA methylation (RdDM) pathway, excluding only PolIV [3•]. Some RdDM mutants had a compromised immune response to pathogenic fungi correlated with a lack of gene induction by JA. In contrast, resistance to a bacterial pathogen was increased, corresponding with elevated levels of salicylic acid-related defense genes and enriched activating chromatin marks H3K4me3 and H3K9ac at the promoter of the SA-inducible gene PR-1. This argues for the overlap between targets of RdDM and SA-signaling and a role of RdDM to relay stress signals to the nucleus.

Stress can certainly induce the production of siRNAs, either via antisense transcription of protein-coding or non-protein-coding sequences, or from inverted repeats. An early example of naturally occurring antisense was the discovery that induction of the Arabidopsis SRO5 expression under salt stress creates a transcript partially complementary to that of the constitutively expressed P5CDH, resulting in dsRNA as a substrate for Dicer-like proteins and siRNAs that are only present and effective under stress [4]. Among 76 long non-protein-coding RNAs (npcRNA) in the Arabidopsis genome, 26 had altered expression levels upon low phosphate, salt or drought stress [5]. Some of them gave rise to 24 bp siRNAs, and npc536 conferred improved root growth under salt stress. By now, many pairs of potential antisense transcripts are identified [6], and natural cis-antisense siRNAs (nat-siRNAs) are defined as a separate class of the small RNA family. Many of them are found exclusively or enriched upon specific stress conditions [7]. One example role of siRNAs in extreme stress tolerance is a dehydration- and ABA-inducible retroelement-derived siRNA that regulates an adaptive response in the resurrection plant

*Craterostigma plantagineum* [8].

Applying tailor-made transcripts of inverted repeats (IRs) is a routine technique to interfere with transcription of target genes with homology to the resulting siRNAs, but similar siRNA can also originate from transcripts of endogenous IRs. Two Arabidopsis repeats, IR71 and IR2039 [9], produce siRNA of different size classes, of which some can silence a GFP-reporter in trans. Endogenous IRs are highly variable in the genome of different ecotypes of Arabidopsis, indicating fast evolution and rapid adaptive changes [9. However, the actual response of IR-derived siRNA to environmental factors and contribution to stress-adaptation is yet to be demonstrated.

Responses of transposable elements (TE) to stress are the topic of reviews by Lisch (this issue) and Bucher et al. (this issue), but TE activation raises the interesting potential of TE-derived small RNAs that target stress-related protein-coding genes [10] and thereby represent an indirect stress signaling pathway.

## Level 2: stress etching on chromatin

Stress signaling leads to stress-adapted gene expression

and also affects chromatin structure at responsive genes, directly or indirectly The changes can affect DNA methylation, histone tail modifications, exchange of histone variants, or nucleosome occupancy and larger chromatin configuration.

# CHAPTER SIX

# •Epigenetic Therapies

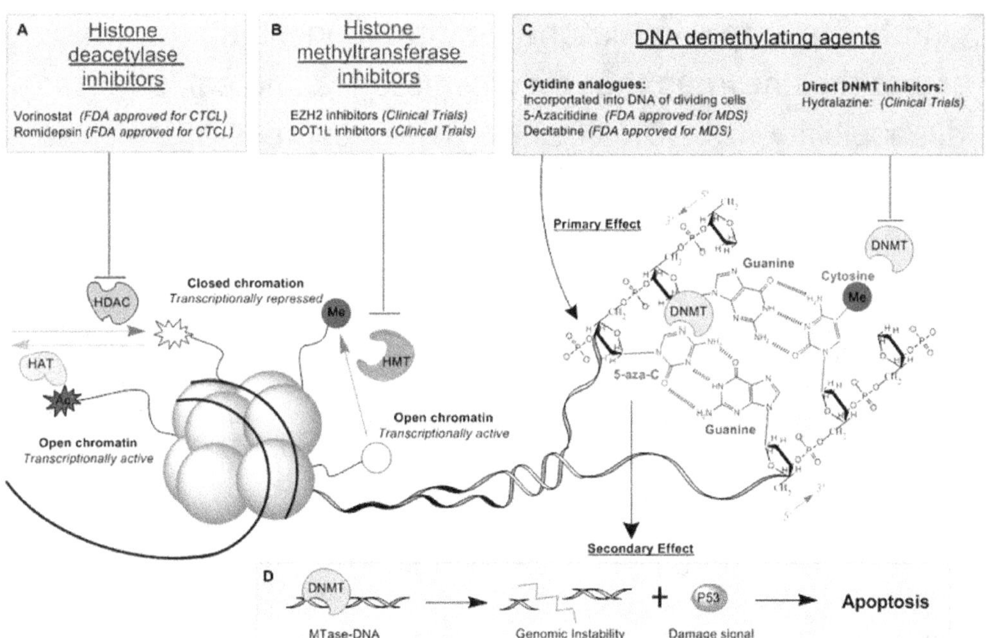



Epigenetic therapies are a new area of research that aims to alter the expression of genes by targeting the mechanisms of epigenetics. The goal of these therapies is to treat or prevent diseases by reversing or preventing the epigenetic changes that contribute to their development.

One example of an epigenetic therapy is the use of drugs that target DNA methylation. These drugs, called demethylating agents, can remove methyl groups from the DNA molecule and reactivate genes that have been suppressed by methylation. This can help to restore normal cellular function and potentially treat diseases caused by abnormal gene expression.

Another example is Histone modification inhibitors, which target the enzymes that modify histones and can alter the accessibility of DNA and gene expression. These inhibitors can help to reactivate genes that have been repressed by histone modification and potentially treat diseases caused by abnormal gene expression.

MicroRNA-targeted therapies are also becoming increasingly popular. These therapies aim to modulate the expression of microRNAs (miRNAs) and their target genes, in order to restore normal cellular function and treat diseases caused by abnormal gene expression.

Overall, epigenetic therapies offer new hope for the treatment of various diseases, including cancer, mental disorders, and cardiovascular diseases. However, more research is needed to fully understand the mechanisms of these therapies and to develop safe and effective drugs.

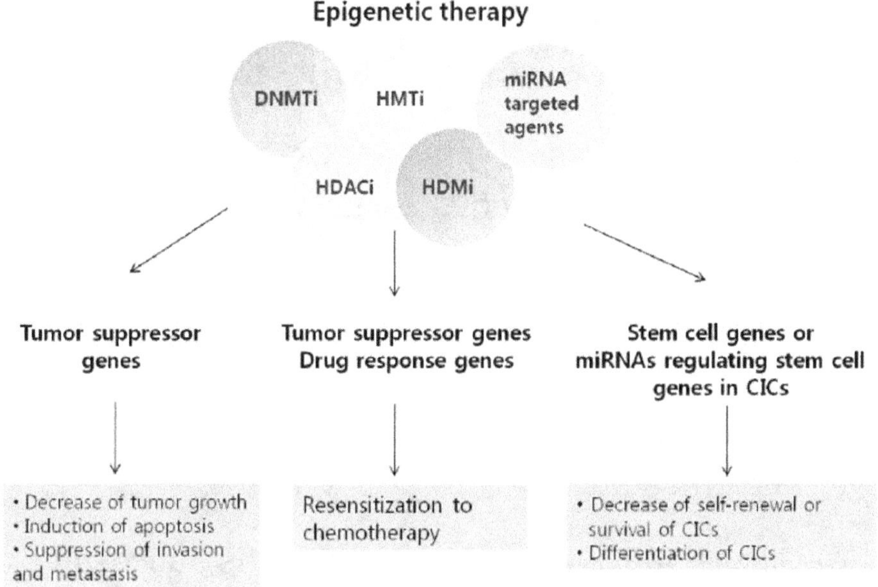


# • Development of epigenetic drugs

The development of epigenetic drugs is a rapidly growing field of research. Scientists are working to design drugs that target the mechanisms of epigenetics in order to treat or prevent a wide range of diseases.

The development of epigenetic drugs can be divided into several stages, including:

1) Identification of potential drug targets: This involves identifying the specific enzymes or proteins

involved in the epigenetic changes that contribute to a particular disease.

2) Drug design and synthesis: Once potential targets have been identified, scientists work to design and synthesize drugs that can specifically bind to and inhibit these targets.

3) Preclinical testing: The drugs are tested in cell culture and animal models to assess their safety and efficacy

4) Clinical trials: If preclinical testing is successful, the drugs are tested in human clinical trials to evaluate their safety and efficacy in treating a specific disease.

5) Approval: If the clinical trials are successful, the drugs are submitted for approval to regulatory agencies such as the FDA.

Currently, several epigenetic drugs are already on the market for the treatment of certain types of cancer, such as azacitidine and decitabine for treating myelodysplastic syndrome, and venetoclax for chronic lymphocytic leukemia, and several other drugs are being tested in clinical trials for the treatment of various diseases such as cancer, mental disorders, and cardiovascular diseases.

Overall, the development of epigenetic drugs is a complex and time-consuming process that requires a significant investment of resources. However, the potential benefits of these drugs in treating a wide range of diseases make it a promising field of research.

# • Epigenetic therapies in clinical trials

Epigenetic therapies are being studied in clinical trials for the treatment of a wide range of diseases, including cancer, mental disorders, and cardiovascular diseases.

In cancer, several epigenetic therapies are already on the market, such as azacitidine and decitabine for treating myelodysplastic syndrome, and venetoclax for chronic lymphocytic leukemia. Other epigenetic drugs for cancer treatment, such as BET inhibitors, HDAC inhibitors and DNA methyltransferase inhibitors, are currently being tested in clinical trials for various types of cancer including lung cancer, prostate cancer, leukemia and lymphoma.

In addition to cancer, epigenetic therapies are also being studied in clinical trials for the treatment of mental disorders such as depression and schizophrenia. For example, HDAC inhibitors are being tested as a potential treatment for depression, while BET inhibitors are being studied as a potential treatment for schizophrenia.

Epigenetic therapies are also being studied in cardiovascular diseases, such as atherosclerosis. For example, drugs that target DNA methylation are being tested as a potential treatment for this disease.

Epigenetic therapies hold great promise as a new class of drugs for the treatment of various diseases. However, more research is needed to fully understand the mechanisms of these therapies and to develop safe and effective drugs

## • Potential future applications

The potential future applications of epigenetic therapies are vast and varied. Here are a few examples of how these therapies may be used in the future:

Cancer treatment: Epigenetic therapies have already shown promise in the treatment of certain types of cancer, such as myelodysplastic syndrome, and chronic lymphocytic leukemia and other types of cancer like lung cancer, prostate cancer, leukemia and lymphoma are currently being studied in clinical trials. With further research, these therapies may become a standard treatment option for a wide range of cancers.

Mental disorders: Epigenetic therapies are currently being

studied in the treatment of mental disorders such as depression and schizophrenia. If successful, these therapies may become a new class of drugs for the treatment of these disorders.

Cardiovascular diseases: Epigenetic therapies are being studied in cardiovascular diseases such as atherosclerosis. If successful, these therapies may become a new treatment option for this disease.

Age-related diseases: Understanding the mechanisms of epigenetic changes in aging may help to develop new strategies for preventing or treating age-related diseases such as Alzheimer's disease and osteoarthritis.

Environmental exposure: Epigenetics plays a role in how environmental exposures affect health. Future therapies may target epigenetic mechanisms to prevent or treat diseases caused by environmental exposures such as pollution and chemicals.

Personalized Medicine: Epigenetic therapies may be used to personalize treatment based on an individual's specific epigenetic profile.

Overall, epigenetic therapies have the potential to revolutionize the way we treat a wide range of diseases, and as research in this field progresses, we can expect to see more therapies developed and more diseases treated with epigenetics in the future.

# CONCLUSION

Summary of key points

Future directions for research

Reference

# • Summary of key points

Epigenetics is the study of changes in gene activity that occur without altering the underlying DNA sequence. These changes can be caused by a variety of factors including environmental exposures, diet and aging. Epigenetics plays a critical role in the development of various diseases such as cancer, mental disorders and cardiovascular diseases.

Epigenetic changes can take many forms, such as DNA methylation, where methyl groups are added to the DNA molecule, leading to suppression of gene expression and changes in cellular function. Histone modification is another form of epigenetics, which occurs when there are changes in the structure of histone proteins that help control gene expression. As we age, these modifications can lead to the repression of certain genes and the activation of others, leading to changes in cellular function and the development of age-related diseases.

Epigenetic therapies are a new area of research that aims to alter the expression of genes by targeting the mechanisms of epigenetics. The goal of these therapies is to treat or prevent diseases by reversing or preventing the epigenetic changes that contribute to their development. Examples of epigenetic therapies include demethylating agents which remove methyl groups from the DNA molecule and reactivate suppressed genes and Histone modification inhibitors that target the enzymes that modify histones and alter gene expression.

The development of epigenetic drugs is a rapidly growing field of research, but it is a complex and time-consuming process. Several epigenetic drugs are already on the market for the treatment of certain types of cancer, and several other drugs are being tested in clinical trials for the treatment of various diseases such as cancer, mental disorders and cardiovascular diseases.

The potential future applications of epigenetic therapies are vast and varied. They have the potential to revolutionize the way we treat a wide range of diseases, and as research in this field progresses, we can expect to see more therapies developed and more diseases treated with epigenetics in the future.

# • Future directions for research

## FUTURE RESEARCH

**Types of future research suggestion**

The Future Research section of your dissertation is often combined with the Research Limitations section of your final, Conclusions chapter. This is because your future research suggestions generally arise out of the research limitations you have identified in your own dissertation. In this article, we discuss six types of future research suggestion. These include: (1) building on a particular finding in your research; (2) addressing a flaw in your research; examining (or testing) a theory (framework or model) either (3) for the first time or (4) in a new context, location and/or culture; (5) re-evaluating and (6) expanding a theory (framework or model). The goal of the article is to help you think about the potential types of future research suggestion that you may want to include in your dissertation.

Before we discuss each of these types of future research suggestion, we should explain why we use the word examining and then put or testing in brackets. This is simply because the word examining may be considered more appropriate when students use a qualitative research design; whereas the word testing fits better with dissertations drawing on a quantitative research design. We also put the words framework or model in brackets after the word theory. We do this because a theory, framework and model are not the same things. In the sections that follow, we discuss six types of future research suggestion.

# Addressing research limitations in your dissertation

In the Research Limitations section of your Conclusions chapter, you will have inevitably detailed the potential flaws (i.e., research limitations) of your dissertation. These may include:

An inability to answer your research questions

Theoretical and conceptual problems

Limitations of your research strategy

Problems of research quality

Identifying what these research limitations were and proposing future research suggestions that address them is arguably the easiest and quickest ways to complete the Future Research section of your Conclusions chapter.

Building on a particular finding or aspect of your research

Often, the findings from your dissertation research will highlight a number of new avenues that could be explored in future studies. These can be grouped into two categories:

### Findings that you did not anticipate

Your dissertation will inevitably lead to findings that you did not anticipate from the start. These are useful when making future research suggestions because they can lead to entirely new avenues to explore in future studies. If this was the case, it is worth (a) briefly describing what these unanticipated findings were and (b) suggesting a research strategy that could be used to explore such findings in future.

### Factors that address unanswered aspects of your research questions

Sometimes, dissertations manage to address all aspects of the research questions that were set. However, this is seldom the case. Typically, there will be aspects of your research questions that could not be answered. This is not necessarily a flaw in your research strategy, but may simply reflect that fact that the findings did not provide all the answers you hoped for. If this was the case, it is worth (a) briefly describing what aspects of your research questions were not answered and (b) suggesting a research strategy that could be used to explore such aspects in future.

### Examining a conceptual framework (or testing a

**theoretical model) for the first time**

You may want to recommend that future research examines the conceptual framework (or tests the theoretical model) that you developed. This is based on the assumption that the primary goal of your dissertation was to set out a conceptual framework (or build a theoretical model). It is also based on the assumption that whilst such a conceptual framework (or theoretical model) was presented, your dissertation did not attempt to examine (or test) it in the field. The focus of your dissertations was most likely a review of the literature rather than something that involved you conducting primary research.

Whilst it is quite rare for dissertations at the undergraduate and master's level to be primarily theoretical in nature like this, it is not unknown. If this was the case, you should think about how the conceptual framework (or theoretical model) that you have presented could be best examined (or tested) in the field. In understanding the how, you should think about two factors in particular:

1. What is the context, location and/or culture that would best lend itself to my conceptual framework (or theoretical model) if it were to be examined (or tested) in the field?

2. What research strategy is most appropriate to examine my conceptual framework (or test my theoretical model)?

If the future research suggestion that you want to make is based on examining your conceptual framework (or testing your theoretical model) in the field, you need to suggest the best scenario for doing so.

## Examining a conceptual framework (or testing a theoretical model) in a new context, location and/or culture

More often than not, you will not only have set out a conceptual framework (or theoretical model), as described in the previous section, but you will also have examined (or tested) it in the field. When you do this, focus is typically placed on a specific context, location and/or culture.

If this is the case, the obvious future research suggestion that you could propose would be to examine your conceptual framework (or test the theoretical model) in a new context, location and/or culture. For example, perhaps you focused on consumers (rather than businesses), or Canada (rather than the United Kingdom), or a more individualistic culture like the United States (rather than a more collectivist culture like China).

When you propose a new context, location and/or culture as your future research suggestion, make sure you justify the choice that you make. For example, there may be little value in future studies looking at different cultures if culture is not an important component underlying your conceptual framework (or theoretical model). If you are not sure whether a new context, location or culture is more appropriate, or what new context, location or culture you should select, a review the literature will often help clarify where you focus should be.

## Expanding a conceptual framework (or theoretical model)

Assuming that you have set out a conceptual framework (or theoretical model) and examined (or tested) it in the field, another series of future research suggestions comes out of expanding that conceptual framework (or theoretical model).

We talk about a series of future research suggestions because there are so many ways that you can expand on your conceptual framework (or theoretical model). For example, you can do this by:

Examining constructs (or variables) that were included in your conceptual framework (or theoretical model) but were not focused.

Looking at a particular relationship aspect of your conceptual framework (or theoretical model) further.

Adding new constructs (or variables) to the conceptual framework (or theoretical model) you set out (if justified by the literature).

It would be possible to include one or a number of these as future research suggestions. Again, make sure that any suggestions you make have are justified, either by your findings or the literature.

## Re-evaluating a conceptual framework (or theoretical model)

With the dissertation process at the undergraduate and master's level lasting between 3 and 9 months, a lot a can happen in between. For example, a specific event (e.g., 9/11, the economic crisis) or some new theory or evidence that undermines (or questions) the literature (theory) and assumptions underpinning your conceptual framework (or theoretical model). Clearly, there is little you can do about this. However, if this happens, reflecting on it and re-evaluating your conceptual framework (or theoretical model), as well as your findings, is an obvious source of future research suggestions.

# ● Reference


1.      Laganà A, Veneziano D, Russo F, Pulvirenti A, Giugno R, Croce CM, Ferro A (2015). "Computational design of artificial RNA molecules for gene regulation". RNA Bioinformatics. Methods in Molecular Biology. Vol. 1269. pp. 393–412. doi:10.1007/978-1-4939-2291-8_25. ISBN 978-1-4939-2290-1. PMC 4425273. PMID 25577393.

2.      Monga I, Qureshi A, Thakur N, Gupta AK, Kumar M (2017). "ASPsiRNA: A Resource of ASP-siRNAs Having Therapeutic Potential for Human Genetic Disorders and Algorithm for Prediction of Their Inhibitory Efficacy". G3: Genes, Genomes, Genetics. 7 (9): 2931–2943. doi:10.1534/g3.117.044024. PMC 5592921. PMID 28696921. CC BY icon.svg Text was copied from this source, which is available under a Creative Commons Attribution 4.0 International License.

9. Brosius J (May 2005). "Waste not, want not--transcript excess in multicellular eukaryotes". Trends in Genetics. 21 (5): 287–8. doi:10.1016/j.tig.2005.02.014. PMID 15851065.

10. Palazzo AF, Lee ES (2015). "Non-coding RNA: what is functional and what is junk?". Frontiers in Genetics. 6: 2. doi:10.3389/fgene.2015.00002. PMC 4306305. PMID 25674102.

11. Mattick, John; Amaral, Paulo (2022). RNA, The Epicenter of Genetic Information : A New Understanding of Molecular Biology. CRC Press. ISBN 9780367623920.

12. Lee, Hyunmin; Zhang, Zhaolei; Krause, Henry M. (December 2019). "Long Noncoding RNAs and Repetitive Elements: Junk or Intimate Evolutionary Partners?". Trends in Genetics. 35 (12): 892–902. doi:10.1016/j.tig.2019.09.006. PMID 31662190. S2CID 204975291.

2. Moore DS (2015). The Developing Genome. Oxford University Press. ISBN 978-0-19-992234-5.[pages needed]

3. Heard E, Martienssen RA (March 2014). "Transgenerational epigenetic inheritance: myths and mechanisms". Cell. 157 (1): 95–109. doi:10.1016/j.cell.2014.02.045. PMC 4020004. PMID 24679529.

3. Jablonka E, Lamb MJ (2010). "Transgenerational epigenetic inheritance.". In Pigliucci M, Müller GB (eds.). Evolution, the expanded synthesis. MIT Press. ISBN 978-0-262-51367-8.

5. Zordan RE, Galgoczy DJ, Johnson AD (August 2006). "Epigenetic properties of white-opaque switching in Candida albicans are based on a self-sustaining transcriptional feedback loop". Proceedings of the National Academy of Sciences of the United States of America. 103 (34): 12807–12812. doi:10.1073/pnas.0605138103. PMC 1535343. PMID 16899543.

6. Beisson J, Sonneborn TM (February 1965). "Cytoplasmic inheritance of the organization of the cell cortex in Paramecium aurelia". Proceedings of the National Academy of Sciences of the United States of America. 53 (2): 275–282. Bibcode:1965PNAS...53..275B. doi:10.1073/pnas.53.2.275. PMC 219507. PMID 14294056.

8. Soto C, Castilla J (July 2004). "The controversial protein-only hypothesis of prion propagation". Nature Medicine. 10 (7): S63–S67. doi:10.1038/nm1069. PMID 15272271. S2CID 8710254.

Vastenhouw NL, Brunschwig K, Okihara KL, Müller F, Tijsterman M, Plasterk RH (August 2006). "Gene expression: long-term gene silencing by RNAi". Nature. 442 (7105): 882. Bibcode:2006Natur.442..882V. doi:10.1038/442882a. PMID 16929289.

Horsthemke B (July 2018). "A critical view on transgenerational epigenetic inheritance in humans". Nature Communications. 9 (1): 2973. Bibcode:2018NatCo...9.2973H. doi:10.1038/s41467-018-05445-5. PMC

6065375. PMID 30061690.

Duclos KK, Hendrikse JL, Jamniczky HA (September 2019). "Investigating the evolution and development of biological complexity under the framework of epigenetics". Evolution & Development. 21 (5): 247–264. doi:10.1111/ede.12301. PMC 6852014. PMID 31268245.

Bond DM, Finnegan EJ (May 2007). "Passing the message on: inheritance of epigenetic traits". Trends in Plant Science. 12 (5): 211–216. doi:10.1016/j.tplants.2007.03.010. PMID 17434332.

Morison IM, Reeve AE (1998). "A catalogue of imprinted genes and parent-of-origin effects in humans and animals". Human Molecular Genetics. 7 (10): 1599–1609. doi:10.1093/hmg/7.10.1599. PMID 9735381.

Scott RJ, Spielman M, Bailey J, Dickinson HG (September 1998). "Parent-of-origin effects on seed development in Arabidopsis thaliana". Development. 125 (17): 3329–3341. doi:10.1242/dev.125.17.3329. PMID 9693137.

Adenot PG, Mercier Y, Renard JP, Thompson EM (November 1997). "Differential H4 acetylation of paternal and maternal chromatin precedes DNA replication and differential transcriptional activity in pronuclei of 1-cell mouse embryos". Development. 124 (22): 4615–4625. doi:10.1242/dev.124.22.4615. PMID 9409678.

Santos F, Hendrich B, Reik W, Dean W (January 2002). "Dynamic reprogramming of DNA methylation in the early mouse embryo". Developmental Biology. 241 (1): 172–182. doi:10.1006/dbio.2001.0501. PMID 11784103.

Oswald J, Engemann S, Lane N, Mayer W, Olek A, Fundele R, et al. (April 2000). "Active demethylation of the paternal genome in the mouse zygote". Current Biology. 10 (8): 475–478. doi:10.1016/S0960-9822(00)00448-6. PMID 10801417.

Fulka H, Mrazek M, Tepla O, Fulka J (December 2004). "DNA methylation pattern in human zygotes and developing embryos". Reproduction. 128 (6): 703–708. doi:10.1530/rep.1.00217. PMID 15579587.

Hackett JA, Sengupta R, Zylicz JJ, Murakami K, Lee C, Down TA, Surani MA (January 2013). "Germline DNA demethylation dynamics and imprint erasure through 5-hydroxymethylcytosine". Science. 339 (6118): 448–452. Bibcode:2013Sci...339..448H. doi:10.1126/science.1229277. PMC 3847602. PMID 23223451.

Surani MA, Hajkova P (2010). "Epigenetic reprogramming of mouse germ cells toward totipotency". Cold Spring Harbor Symposia on Quantitative Biology. 75: 211–218. doi:10.1101/sqb.2010.75.010. PMID 21139069.

Zhang Z, Shibahara K, Stillman B (November 2000). "PCNA connects DNA replication to epigenetic inheritance in yeast". Nature. 408 (6809): 221–225. Bibcode:2000Natur.408..221Z. doi:10.1038/35041601. PMID 11089978. S2CID 205010657.

Henderson DS, Banga SS, Grigliatti TA, Boyd JB (March 1994). "Mutagen sensitivity and suppression of position-effect variegation result from mutations in mus209, the Drosophila gene encoding PCNA". The EMBO Journal. 13 (6): 1450–1459. doi:10.1002/j.1460-2075.1994.tb06399.x. PMC 394963. PMID 7907981.

Probst AV, Dunleavy E, Almouzni G (March 2009). "Epigenetic inheritance during the cell cycle". Nature Reviews. Molecular Cell Biology. 10 (3): 192–206. doi:10.1038/nrm2640. PMID 19234478. S2CID 205494340.

Morgan HD, Santos F, Green K, Dean W, Reik W (April 2005). "Epigenetic reprogramming in mammals". Human Molecular Genetics. 14 (Review Issue 1): R47–R58. doi:10.1093/hmg/ddi114. PMID 15809273.

Santos F, Peters AH, Otte AP, Reik W, Dean W (April 2005). "Dynamic chromatin modifications characterise the first cell cycle in mouse embryos". Developmental Biology. 280 (1): 225–236.

doi:10.1016/j.ydbio.2005.01.025. PMID 15766761.

Taguchi YH (2015). "Identification of aberrant gene expression associated with aberrant promoter methylation in primordial germ cells between E13 and E16 rat F3 generation vinclozolin lineage". BMC Bioinformatics. 16 (Suppl 18): S16. doi:10.1186/1471-2105-16-S18-S16. PMC 4682393. PMID 26677731.

Richards EJ (May 2006). "Inherited epigenetic variation--revisiting soft inheritance". Nature Reviews. Genetics. 7 (5): 395–401. doi:10.1038/nrg1834. PMID 16534512. S2CID 21961242.

Jablonka E, Lamb MJ (1998). "Epigenetic inheritance in evolution". Journal of Evolutionary Biology. 11 (2): 159–183. doi:10.1046/j.1420-9101.1998.11020159.x. S2CID 55965463.

Bird A, Kirschner M, Gerhart J, Moore T, Wopert L (1998). "Comments on "Epigenetic inheritance in evolution"". Journal of Evolutionary Biology. 11 (2): 185–188, 213–217, 229–232, 239–240. doi:10.1046/j.1420-9101.1998.11020185.x.

Jablonka E, Raz G (June 2009). "Transgenerational epigenetic inheritance: prevalence, mechanisms, and implications for the study of heredity and evolution". The Quarterly Review of Biology. 84 (2): 131–176. CiteSeerX 10.1.1.617.6333. doi:10.1086/598822. PMID 19606595. S2CID 7233550.

Rassoulzadegan M, Cuzin F (April 2015). "Epigenetic heredity: RNA-mediated modes of phenotypic variation". Annals of the New York Academy of Sciences. 1341 (1): 172–175. Bibcode:2015NYASA1341..172R. doi:10.1111/nyas.12694. PMID 25726734. S2CID 23244919.

Bossdorf O, Richards CL, Pigliucci M (February 2008). "Epigenetics for ecologists". Ecology Letters. 11 (2): 106–115. doi:10.1111/j.1461-0248.2007.01130.x. PMID 18021243.

Molinier J, Ries G, Zipfel C, Hohn B (August 2006). "Transgeneration memory of stress in plants". Nature. 442 (7106): 1046–1049. Bibcode:2006Natur.442.1046M. doi:10.1038/nature05022. PMID 16892047. S2CID 4329910.

Coe EH (June 1959). "A regular and continuing conversion-type phenomenon at the B locus in maize". Proceedings of the National Academy of Sciences of the United States of America. 45 (6): 828–832. Bibcode:1959PNAS...45..828C. doi:10.1073/pnas.45.6.828. PMC 222644. PMID 16590451.

Chandler VL (February 2007). "Paramutation: from maize to mice". Cell. 128 (4): 641–645. doi:10.1016/j.cell.2007.02.007. PMID 17320501.

Stam M, Belele C, Ramakrishna W, Dorweiler JE, Bennetzen JL, Chandler VL (October 2002). "The regulatory regions required for B' paramutation and expression are located far upstream of the maize b1 transcribed sequences". Genetics. 162 (2): 917–930. doi:10.1093/genetics/162.2.917. PMC 1462281. PMID 12399399.

Belele CL, Sidorenko L, Stam M, Bader R, Arteaga-Vazquez MA, Chandler VL (2013-10-17). "Specific tandem repeats are sufficient for paramutation -induced trans-generational silencing". PLOS Genetics. 9 (10): e1003773. doi:10.1371/journal.pgen.1003773. PMC 3798267. PMID 24146624.

Arteaga-Vazquez M, Sidorenko L, Rabanal FA, Shrivistava R, Nobuta K, Green PJ, et al. (July 2010). "RNA-mediated trans-communication can establish paramutation at the b1 locus in maize". Proceedings of the National Academy of Sciences of the United States of America. 107 (29): 12986–12991. Bibcode:2010PNAS..10712986A. doi:10.1073/pnas.1007972107. PMC 2919911. PMID 20616013.

Louwers M, Bader R, Haring M, van Driel R, de Laat W, Stam M (March 2009). "Tissue- and expression level-specific chromatin looping at maize b1 epialleles". The Plant Cell. 21 (3): 832–842. doi:10.1105/tpc.108.064329. PMC 2671708. PMID 19336692.

Haring M, Bader R, Louwers M, Schwabe A, van Driel R, Stam M (August 2010). "The role of DNA methylation, nucleosome occupancy and histone modifications in paramutation". The Plant Journal. 63 (3): 366–378. doi:10.1111/j.1365-313X.2010.04245.x. PMID 20444233.

Dorweiler JE, Carey CC, Kubo KM, Hollick JB, Kermicle JL, Chandler VL (November 2000). "mediator of paramutation1 is required for establishment and maintenance of paramutation at multiple maize loci". The Plant Cell. 12 (11): 2101–2118. doi:10.1105/tpc.12.11.2101. PMC 150161. PMID 11090212.

Chandler V, Alleman M (April 2008). "Paramutation: epigenetic instructions passed across generations". Genetics. 178 (4): 1839–1844. doi:10.1093/genetics/178.4.1839. PMC 2323780. PMID 18430919.

Nobuta K, Lu C, Shrivastava R, Pillay M, De Paoli E, Accerbi M, et al. (September 2008). "Distinct size distribution of endogeneous siRNAs in maize: Evidence from deep sequencing in the mop1-1 mutant". Proceedings of the National Academy of Sciences of the United States of America. 105 (39): 14958–14963. Bibcode:2008PNAS..10514958N. doi:10.1073/pnas.0808066105. PMC 2567475. PMID 18815367.

Alleman M, Sidorenko L, McGinnis K, Seshadri V, Dorweiler JE, White J, et al. (July 2006). "An RNA-dependent RNA polymerase is required for paramutation in maize". Nature. 442 (7100): 295–298. Bibcode:2006Natur.442..295A. doi:10.1038/nature04884. PMID 16855589. S2CID 4419412.

Arteaga-Vazquez MA, Chandler VL (April 2010). "Paramutation in maize: RNA mediated trans-generational gene silencing". Current Opinion in Genetics & Development. 20 (2): 156–163. doi:10.1016/j.gde.2010.01.008. PMC 2859986. PMID 20153628.

Huang J, Lynn JS, Schulte L, Vendramin S, McGinnis K (2017-01-01). "Epigenetic Control of Gene Expression in Maize". International Review of Cell and Molecular Biology. 328: 25–48.

doi:10.1016/bs.ircmb.2016.08.002. ISBN 9780128122204. PMID 28069135.

Chandler VL (October 2010). "Paramutation's properties and puzzles". Science. 330 (6004): 628–629. Bibcode:2010Sci...330..628C. doi:10.1126/science.1191044. PMID 21030647. S2CID 13248794.

Zheng X, Chen L, Xia H, Wei H, Lou Q, Li M, et al. (January 2017). "Transgenerational epimutations induced by multi-generation drought imposition mediate rice plant's adaptation to drought condition". Scientific Reports. 7: 39843. Bibcode:2017NatSR...739843Z. doi:10.1038/srep39843. PMC 5209664. PMID 28051176.

Rasmann S, De Vos M, Casteel CL, Tian D, Halitschke R, Sun JY, et al. (February 2012). "Herbivory in the previous generation primes plants for enhanced insect resistance". Plant Physiology. 158 (2): 854–863. doi:10.1104/pp.111.187831. PMC 3271773. PMID 22209873.

Quadrana L, Colot V (November 2016). "Plant Transgenerational Epigenetics". Annual Review of Genetics. 50 (1): 467–491. doi:10.1146/annurev-genet-120215-035254. PMID 27732791.

Duszynska D, Vilhjalmsson B, Castillo Bravo R, Swamidatta S, Juenger TE, Donoghue MT, et al. (September 2019). "Transgenerational effects of inter-ploidy cross direction on reproduction and F2 seed development of Arabidopsis thaliana F1 hybrid triploids". Plant Reproduction. 32 (3): 275–289. doi:10.1007/s00497-019-00369-6. PMC 6675909. PMID 30903284.

Wei Y, Schatten H, Sun QY (2014). "Environmental epigenetic inheritance through gametes and implications for human reproduction". Human Reproduction Update. 21 (2): 194–208. doi:10.1093/humupd/dmu061. PMID 25416302.

Lalande M (1996). "Parental imprinting and human disease". Annual Review of Genetics. 30: 173–195. doi:10.1146/annurev.genet.30.1.173.

PMID 8982453.

da Cruz, R. S., Chen, E., Smith, M., Bates, J., & de Assis, S. (2020). Diet and Transgenerational Epigenetic Inheritance of Breast Cancer: The Role of the Paternal Germline. Frontiers in nutrition, 7, 93. https://doi.org/10.3389/fnut.2020.0009

Fontelles CC, Carney E, Clarke J, Nguyen NM, Yin C, Jin L, Cruz MI, Ong TP, Hilakivi-Clarke L, de Assis S (June 2016). "Paternal overweight is associated with increased breast cancer risk in daughters in a mouse model". Scientific Reports. 6: 28602. Bibcode:2016NatSR...628602F. doi:10.1038/srep28602. PMC 4919621. PMID 27339599.

Napoli C, Benincasa G, Loscalzo J (April 2019). "Epigenetic Inheritance Underlying Pulmonary Arterial Hypertension". Arteriosclerosis, Thrombosis, and Vascular Biology. 39 (4): 653–664. doi:10.1161/ATVBAHA.118.312262. PMC 6436974. PMID 30727752.

Weaver IC, Cervoni N, Champagne FA, D'Alessio AC, Sharma S, Seckl JR, et al. (August 2004). "Epigenetic programming by maternal behavior". Nature Neuroscience. 7 (8): 847–854. doi:10.1038/nn1276. PMID 15220929. S2CID 1649281.

McGowan PO, Sasaki A, D'Alessio AC, Dymov S, Labonté B, Szyf M, et al. (March 2009). "Epigenetic regulation of the glucocorticoid receptor in human brain associates with childhood abuse". Nature Neuroscience. 12 (3): 342–348. doi:10.1038/nn.2270. PMC 2944040. PMID 19234457.

Meaney MJ, Szyf M (2005). "Environmental programming of stress responses through DNA methylation: life at the interface between a dynamic environment and a fixed genome". Dialogues in Clinical Neuroscience. 7 (2): 103–123. doi:10.31887/DCNS.2005.7.2/mmeaney. PMC 3181727. PMID 16262207.

Radtke KM, Ruf M, Gunter HM, Dohrmann K, Schauer M, Meyer A, Elbert T (July 2011). "Transgenerational impact of intimate partner violence on methylation in the promoter of the glucocorticoid receptor". Translational Psychiatry. 1 (July 19): e21. doi:10.1038/tp.2011.21. PMC 3309516. PMID 22832523.

Kioumourtzoglou MA, Coull BA, O'Reilly ÉJ, Ascherio A, Weisskopf MG (July 2018). "Association of Exposure to Diethylstilbestrol During Pregnancy With Multigenerational Neurodevelopmental Deficits". JAMA Pediatrics. 172 (7): 670–677. doi:10.1001/jamapediatrics.2018.0727. PMC 6137513. PMID 29799929.

MedlinePlus. Degenerative Nerve Diseases.

Gitler AD, Dhillon P, Shorter J. Neurodegenerative disease: models, mechanisms, and a new hope. Disease Models & Mechanisms. 2017;10(5):499-502.

Levenson RW, Sturm VE, Haase CM. Emotional and behavioral symptoms in neurodegenerative disease: A model for studying the neural bases of psychopathology. Annu Rev Clin Psychol. 2014;10:581-606.

Sheinerman KS, Umansky SR. Early detection of neurodegenerative diseases. Cell Cycle. 2013;12(1):1-2.

Frontiers for Young Minds. Why Doesn't Your Brain Heal Like Your Skin?.

Peters R. Ageing and the brain. Postgrad Med J. 2006;82(964):84-88. doi:10.1136/pgmj.2005.036665

Armstrong R. What causes neurodegenerative disease? Folia Neuropatholgica. 2020;58(2):93-112.

Price DL, Sisodia SS, Borchelt DR. Genetic neurodegenerative diseases: the human illness and transgenic models. Science. 1998;282(5391):1079–1083.

Spires-Jones TL, Attems J, Thal DR. Interactions of pathological proteins in neurodegenerative diseases. Acta Neuropathol. 2017;134(2):187-205.

Brown RC, Lockwood AH, Sonawane BR. Neurodegenerative diseases: an overview of environmental risk factors. Environ Health Perspect. 2005;113(9):1250-1256.

Alzheimer's Association. 2022 Alzheimer's disease Facts and Figures.

National Institute on Aging. What Are the Signs of Alzheimer's Disease?.

National Institute on Aging. What Causes Alzheimer's Disease?.

National Institute of Neurological Disorders and Stroke. Amyotrophic lateral sclerosis (ALS) fact sheet.

National Library of Medicine. Huntington's Disease.

National Institute on Aging. What is Lewy body dementia? Causes, symptoms, and treatments.

National Institute on Aging. Parkinson's Disease: causes, symptoms, and treatments.


Kiaei M. New hopes and challenges for treatment of neurodegenerative disorders: great opportunities for young neuroscientists. Basic Clin Neurosci. 2013;4(1):3-4.


99. Vaquero A , Scher M , Lee D , Erdjument-Bromage H , Tempst P , Reinberg D. Human SirT1 interacts with histone H1 and promotes formation of facultative heterochromatin. Mol Cell 16: 93– 105, 2004.

Crossref | PubMed | ISI | Google Scholar  100.  Veurink M , Koster M , Berg LT. The history of DES, lessons to be learned. Pharm World Sci 27: 139– 143, 2005.

Crossref | Google Scholar  101.  Villar-Garea A , Esteller M. Histone deacetylase inhibitors: understanding a new wave of anticancer agents. Int J Cancer 112: 171– 178, 2004.

Crossref | ISI | Google Scholar  102.  Villar-Garea A , Fraga MF , Espada J , Esteller M. Procaine is a DNA-demethylating agent with growth-inhibitory effects in human cancer cells. Cancer Res 63: 4984– 4989, 2003.

ISI | Google Scholar  103.  Vogt G , Huber M , Thiemann M , van den Boogaart G , Schmitz OJ , Schubart CD. Production of different phenotypes from the same genotype in the same environment by developmental variation. J Exp Biol 211: 510– 523, 2008.

Crossref | PubMed | ISI | Google Scholar  104.  Waddington CH. The epigenotype. Endeavour 1: 18– 20, 1942.

Google Scholar  105.  Warri A , Saarinen NM , Makela S , Hilakivi-Clarke L. The role of early life genistein exposures in modifying breast cancer risk. Br J Cancer 98: 1485– 1493, 2008.

Crossref | ISI | Google Scholar  106.  Waterland RA. Assessing the effects of high methionine intake on DNA methylation. J Nutr 136: 1706S– 1710S, 2006.

Crossref | ISI | Google Scholar  107.  Waterland RA. Do maternal methyl supplements in mice affect DNA methylation of offspring? J Nutr 133: 238; author reply 239, 2003.

Crossref | ISI | Google Scholar  108.  Waterland RA , Dolinoy DC , Lin JR , Smith CA , Shi X , Tahiliani KG. Maternal methyl supplements increase offspring DNA methylation at axin fused. Genesis 44: 401– 406, 2006.

Crossref | PubMed | ISI | Google Scholar  109.  Waterland RA , Travisano

M , Tahiliani KG , Rached MT , Mirza S. Methyl donor supplementation prevents transgenerational amplification of obesity. Int J Obes (Lond) 32: 1373– 1379, 2008.

Crossref | ISI | Google Scholar  110.  Whitelaw NC , Whitelaw E. How lifetimes shape epigenotype within and across generations. Hum Mol Genet 15, Spec No 2: R131– 137, 2006.

Crossref | ISI | Google Scholar  111.  Wilson VL , Jones PA. DNA methylation decreases in aging but not in immortal cells. Science 220: 1055– 1057, 1983.

Crossref | PubMed | ISI | Google Scholar  112.  Wilson VL , Smith RA , Ma S , Cutler RG. Genomic 5-methyldeoxycytidine decreases with age. J Biol Chem 262: 9948– 9951, 1987.

PubMed | ISI | Google Scholar  113.  Xiang N , Zhao R , Song G , Zhong W. Selenite reactivates silenced genes by modifying DNA methylation and histones in prostate cancer cells. Carcinogenesis 29: 2175– 2181, 2008.

Crossref | ISI | Google Scholar  114.  Yenbutr P , Hilakivi-Clarke L , Passaniti A. Hypomethylation of an exon I estrogen receptor CpG island in spontaneous and carcinogen-induced mammary tumorigenesis in the rat. Mech Ageing Dev 106: 93– 102, 1998.

Crossref | ISI | Google Scholar

www.ingramcontent.com/pod-product-compliance
Lightning Source LLC
Chambersburg PA
CBHW071218260726

48653CB00042B/1253